Be You- T - Full:

Looking your best with Botox, lasers and other magical cosmetic treatments

Enjoy!
Beth Haney

Dr. Beth Haney, DNP

2012

Library of Congress Cataloging-in-Publication Data
ISBN #: 978-0-9859203-1-9 (alk. paper)

BE YOU-T-FULL:
Looking your best with Botox, lasers
and other magical cosmetic treatments

Edited by Lisa Hart
Illustrations by Ross Loehner

Printed in United States of America
Paperback

Library of Congress Control Number: 20 12 91 35 82

www.beyoutfull.net
www.luxemedspa.net

formation on how to care for your skin, prevent further amage and perhaps look a little fresher. It will surely be omething I'll recommend for my patients."

Kristin Rhodes, FNP, Family Nurse Practitioner

"Be You-T-Full is very informative and fun to ead! I recommend it to my patients because it explains omplex procedures and treatments in an easy to nderstand way. They will have a clear idea of what they vant or need and what really works! It also answers uestions about regular skin care issues for those who on't necessarily want to get cosmetic treatments done."

JoAnn Eastman, RN, BSN, Aesthetic Specialist

"After months of fretting about the lines going cross my forehead, by my nose and mouth as well as the ittle wrinkles around my eyes- I went for my first onsultation and treatments. I was lucky to be in the ands of a trusted expert who told me what my options were. I have been pleased with the results and feel that it has taken years off my appearance. This book clearly explains what can and can't be accomplished by various treatments available. It's valuable for anyone interested in preserving or renewing his or her appearance."

- Theresa Ullrich, FNP, aesthetic patient and Family Nurse Practitioner

Read what others are saying about Be You
Looking your best with Botox, lasers, and o
cosmetic treatments

"There has been a veritable explosion
and aesthetic therapies that have come to m
last decade or so. As a nurse practitioner, pati
for advice and want to know what "really"
Haney uses a humorous and easy-to-understa
writing directed to consumers, to describe t
aesthetic options. I will recommend Be You
both men and women who want more infor
they can make informed choices and continu
their best through-out life!"

- Dr. Susan Tiso, DNP, Doctor of Nursing Practice
Clinical Professor - University of California, Irvine

"I have been seeing Beth for over 5 years
always has the most up to date lasers available an
love about her is she always strives for a natui
Having cystic acne in my past, my skin depends c
keep it looking the best and this book is like h
thorough consultation with her and it makes
skincare easy to understand."

- Vicki Gunvalson, star of Real Housewives of Orange
County

"Every person deserves a consultation with
expert, such as Dr. Haney and this is it. Her book
like a group of friends sitting around a party discu
skin care with her, but getting correct, clinically ev

"I have been getting Botox and fillers for years and cannot imagine life without these great treatments! I read Be You-T-Full and now understand what the best options are for me to stay as young looking as possible. People tell me all the time that I look like I'm 30! I recently had a laser resurfacing treatment and after a couple of weeks, I saw a huge difference in my skin - so much smoother but still natural looking. I am so thankful I won't need to have a facelift any time soon!"

- Patty, 48-year old aesthetic patient

Table of Contents

Dedication

This book is dedicated to all the people who have entered my life, both briefly and lasting. Each person has taught me something along the way. I hope I have given back something of meaning to those who have and will attend my classes, enter my treatment room, or read this book. Of course, this dedication would not be complete without acknowledging my wonderful husband whose amazing support is an incredible gift and I am so honored to be able to share my life with him.

And last (but not least!), to all of the patients who looked in the mirror after we completed a treatment and said, "WOW!" You all have "made my day" countless times and transformed my job into the most rewarding experience anyone could ask for.

I am forever grateful.

Thank you to each one of you.

Acknowledgements

I believe that successful people do not work alone; there are always people who support, assist, and encourage them from the sidelines. Therefore it is with utmost gratitude that I thank the following people for their help in making the dream of this book a reality for me.

Thank you to my editor Lisa Hart, for her keen eye, perseverance and attention to detail. I am so fortunate that our paths crossed years ago. To Ross Loehner, for his incredible artistic gift, patience and creativity with the illustrations. To my manager, Nichole Ullrich. Her dedication to my aesthetic practice, allowed me to steal away to write, knowing the office would run smoothly.

Thanks to Nickie Schalliol and Jenna Norwood for their young eyes and millennial age viewpoints. To Donna Clawson, Mary Gentry and Surani Hayre-Kwan for their honest input and unconditional support. To Susan Tiso, Susie Phillips, Karen Deck, and Camille Fitzpatrick, for their love and encouragement (and strong opinions about the cover). To Ric Franzi: who mentored me in the beginning of this endeavor and guided me on the right path to becoming an author.

Thank you to everyone.

Foreword

Dr. WILL KIRBY - Board Certified Dermatologist, Fellow, American Osteopathic College of Dermatology; Medical Director, Dr. Tattoff, Inc., Clinical Assistant Professor of Dermatology, Western University of Health Sciences, Clinical Assistant Professor, Division of Dermatology, Nova Southeastern University.

Aesthetics is a complex world intertwined with the perceived standards of beauty created by society that integrates aspects of health and wellness. While everyone has a different definition of health and beauty, one thing is universally common: "These days, people not only want to *be* healthy they also want to *look* healthy". Resultantly, aesthetic treatments have grown to become commonplace however significant confusion remains and obtaining accurate and honest information persists. I am thrilled that Beth has taken initiative to provide patients and health care providers alike a guide to navigate the aesthetic waters.

Followed closely by choosing effective products and aesthetic services, understanding how your skin works is the first and most important step in looking great. It is all too easy to get lost in the quagmire of advertising, inaccurate internet information and suspicious product claims but this book makes skin and aesthetic options much easier to understand, so that you can create your own strategy for looking your best.

The information herein provides the reader a wealth of tools they can use when seeking aesthetic treatment and allows them to make more informed decisions about their cosmetic care. Moreover, anyone who is interested in achieving their best look *without* visiting an office for treatments will also find pearls of information contained in these pages. Beth provides immediately useful and timely tips on some of the best skin care options for a diverse population and I recommend this book to men and women of all backgrounds and ages as well as clinicians interested in gaining a deeper understanding of aesthetic medicine. By following the advice found here you can lay the foundation for healthy and radiant skin for years to come with the ultimate goal of helping you look as good as you feel!

Important Message to the Reader

This book was written to offer you - the reader, information on current treatments, procedures, and product ingredients to look your best, and help you put the brakes on aging (It's inevitable that we will all get older but none of us want to *look* or *feel* older!). These pages are not meant to replace an in-depth consultation with your aesthetic provider and it is highly recommended you receive a thorough consultation before you undergo any cosmetic treatment. The author and any individual involved with the writing of this book, expressly disclaims any responsibility for any negative outcomes that result from the use of the information included within these pages. This book contains general information and is not to be a substitute for nursing or medical advice. The intent of this book is to provide you with information you can understand and communicate easily with an aesthetic provider; then by working together, reach your desired beauty goals.

Introduction

For many of us, the media continues to define unattainable standards of beauty through glossy magazine covers, movie content, and television programs. Bedeviling, yes. Subsequently, the demand for aesthetic medical treatments continues to grow at a rapid pace, not just in the United States but globally. Most people want to look and stay "young-looking" for as long as they can. The combination of the media and our desire to be young forever feeds this frenzy and creates a lot of questions.

This is not a how-to book written by celebrities – it's a no-nonsense guide to use in whatever way is appropriate for you. It is a compilation of real techniques, skin care options, and medical aesthetic (visually appealing) treatments that are effective for many people. Men included!

Finances or aesthetic desire should be taken into consideration, however there are options available that are less expensive and will be of benefit to you and your appearance. Specific surgical treatments, surgical recommendations and make-up ingredients will not be included but what will be included are un-biased opinions and facts about some fantastic downright magical treatments including Botox, Restylane, laser treatments, peels, and many more!

Thoughtful suggestions based on many years of experience, both in providing and receiving these treatments as well as review of the literature, are contained within these pages. After reading through this book you will have the knowledge and information to enhance and maintain your appearance for many years to come. Oh, but guess what! You will also be armed with the basic understanding of skin care product ingredients and future treatments. *Be You-T-Full* is intended for all men and women; all shapes, sizes and ages, whether you're a sun worshiper, sun phobic, product-a-holic or needle phobic. It will open your eyes to what really works and what doesn't. Beauty has no limits!

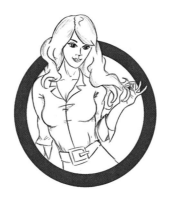

Chapter 1

HOW DOES SHE LOOK SO YOUNG?

Secrets

Have you ever wondered what you could do to look better? Or wondered why some people seem to look *better* as they age? Have you thought about going to a medical spa or plastic surgeon's office to find out what you can do and then, at the last minute, you chicken out? You're just too embarrassed or nervous to talk to someone about what's been bugging you about your appearance? Or maybe you thought you'd have to take a second mortgage out on your house…or maybe you thought you'd look like a puffy balloon face when you were done with your cosmetic binge. Well, this book will help unlock the secrets and guide you savvy girls (and boys) through this crazy maze of cosmetic treatments.

Be You-T-Full is filled with real ideas, solutions, and *answers* to how and why so many women are beautiful on the inside and out, and how you can be too. Yes, genetics have something to do with how you look, bone structure, eyebrow placement (sort of), lips, shape of your face, as well as body type. Now you can do something to enhance your God-given looks. As we have learned, most beautiful women don't just offer their secrets to anyone who asks, they prefer to keep their "secrets" to themselves or they'll fib a little and say it's this fabulous night cream they found or this supplement they take to keep them looking young – Ha! Well, here is one little secret: – most of us are *not* born beautiful or up to the standards society has categorized as beautiful. Being beautiful isn't just about what's on the outside, its what's on the inside that matters too. Whether you were born beautiful or not, rest assured you'll find some gems here that you will think were written just for you!

Women who are lucky enough to grow up beautiful and stay that way very often enhance their appearance in some form or another, either surgically or non-surgically. On a regular basis, I see beautiful women all day long who say they absolutely "can't live without _____" (you can fill in the blank with Botox, Dysport, Juvederm, and so on). It's not a big surprise but more and more men are also getting these non-surgical treatments done!

One of the many reasons more and more men and women are getting these magical treatments are because the results are natural, noticeable, and truly make the face more youthful without changing the appearance too much. We still want to look like ourselves – just BETTER! We want people to comment on how great we look and ask, "What are you doing? You look fabulous!" We *don't* want people to say "What happened?" or "What did you do to your face?" Of course, we have all seen celebrities that make us wonder 'Doesn't she look in the mirror?' or 'Who would do that to her?' Even some men make headlines when they have gone too far or have had a procedure done that is too obvious.

The secret is to be subtle. In the early days of aesthetic treatments, we didn't really have too many choices. Collagen and facelifts were about it, one extreme to the other. Collagen still only lasts about 3-months, requiring constant office visits for touch ups. Hopefully if someone got treated with Collagen, they would come out unscathed (not bruised) so they could go out in public soon after treatment. And facelifts – whoa! Usually women would wait until their face had drooped and dropped pretty badly before they would opt for this surgery. Then what did you have? A yanked or pulled face. That's right, get- it- up- there! Crank-it-up…Youth used to be associated with pulling everything upwards and onwards – heave ho! Today, after wondering for so long if there was a better way, we have figured out something ideal called fullness.

Yes, fullness is more youthful than pulled. Have you ever really looked at a young face? There's fullness in the cheeks, lips, temples, and jawline. Now we're not talking about fullness like a 10-month old baby – that would look ridiculous on a woman in her 40's or 50's. You don't want to look like a balloon on a stick. But unfortunately, this is what happens when people get a bit carried away – more fullness is better, right? Like let's keep going until it explodes! Wrong.

Self-restraint is key for both patient and practitioner. If one has it and the other doesn't, the scenario can go like this: the patient is dying for her lips to be so big, she can't close her mouth and the practitioner makes it happen – oh boy. I'll bet people ask Lips La-Rue where she gets her lips done and then head the other direction. Good idea? Yes! This is an example of no self-restraint on either side. One-sided willpower can look like a woman with cheeks so full they distort her eyes or have her eyebrows and forehead frozen into place. Mad? Sad? Glad? People will ask Zip Lock what happened to her face, if they comment at all – scary. The patient or practitioner, or both can be to blame for this scenario. See the problem here? Thought you would.

Assignment: Take a look in the mirror and try and figure out what you would like to improve, sometimes it's hard to pin point, you just don't like what you see. This is where an expert comes in and helps. Find an office where you feel comfortable and the practitioner takes time with you to help you

discover what will work best for your concerns. This is very important. You want to make decisions regarding your transformation with your practitioner. Suggestions are always nice. The practitioner you choose should have a lot of experience and education, one you trust based on your specific issues. You only have one face and no one else has it, it's yours exclusively. Hoorah!

On the other hand, you do NOT want someone to tell you what you need to do. If the mole in the center of your forehead with the black curly hair growing out of it didn't bother you and your practitioner suggested to get rid of it, you might spend $500 or more on something you didn't really care about in the first place. How would that feel? Now, if your hollow cheeks are bothering you and you decide with your practitioner you would like them more youthful, then fill'er up! You'll love the results and it will be money well spent – right? If you want that little magical eyebrow lift that Botox gives you and your practitioner offers you that wonderful lifted look, you experience sheer bliss right? The point is if you want to be happy, you need to know what you want to improve, for you, yourself. However, you can count on your experienced practitioner to give you advice, recommendations, and help you be your best.

These treatments can help uplift your spirit, help you feel better, and help you love the way you look. Many people, who have been receiving aesthetic treatments regularly, look younger and more rested than they did 10 years ago! Let's call these people "new natural beauties or NNBs". This is not saying you have to be in the office getting touch-ups every week, but regular maintenance, like getting your hair styled or going to the gym, makes a difference in your appearance. Depending on your unique concerns, you might be in the office anywhere from once a month for microdermabrasions to once a year or even longer for laser treatments (more on these treatments in the following chapters).

Many NNBs say they run into friends they haven't seen in months or years and their friends exclaim "Wow, you look great!" or "What are you doing to look so young?" or "How come I'm aging and you're not?" If you want to see some amazing results, try a treatment or two (or three) and then compare your driver's license or passport photos from before you started getting treatments to your current photo. The proof is in the pudding, chocolate please...

Welcome to the Club

We've all had fears of trying something new, a new recipe, a new hairstylist, a new boyfriend, a new job, or a new way of doing something. We might think, "What if it doesn't work? What if I really screw up and tell them the wrong thing? What if I love the new way and totally abandon my old way? What will my friends/family say?" Or in the case of Botox or the other magical cosmetic treatments, "What if I fall in love with it?" Well...here's a story that might ease your mind.

Recently, a patient said, "I want you to know, my husband totally loves his Botox! He is worse than me now about wanting to get in here for his next treatment!" This is remarkable because this woman had to drag her husband into the office for his first treatment. There he sat, feigning ease with an occasional joke about vanity or needles. He was very rugged, tanned, and macho so he couldn't show any anxiety about getting this treatment – he wasn't scared, he's not scared "a'nuthin", but the beads of sweat on his brow said something else. Hey, not only that, but what would the guys think if they knew he was here for this? Newsflash! His buddies come in too but we can't tell him because of the extreme confidential nature of this medical business. (Don't be shocked. Half of your friends are doing it too). Ah, such is life.

His wife sat back and reveled in the thought of her husband squirming in the chair, about to receive his first glimpse into the private world of "The Club" as we tend to call it. Yes dahling, welcome to the Club. Anyone can join but once you're in, it's hard to get out. Of course, you can always exit the Club but you'll never want to, because the results are marvelous and you will look fabulous, but in a natural, not phony-baloney way.

Confidence

Another attribute of beautiful women like yourself is the feeling of self-confidence, knowing who you are and loving it! You're fabulous and you know it – clap your hands. Now go stand in front of that dreadful full-length mirror and say these magical words "I'm fabulous!" Now, wasn't that easy? I'll bet you felt like a numbskull doing that little exercise. Don't worry, you'll get used to it, especially when all of your friends, family, and co-workers are saying, "Wow, you're fabulous!" to you too. You see, all the latest women's magazines and articles you're reading tout the benefits of being confident.

There are reasons for this, confidence makes you stand up straighter, speak more clearly, and survey your surroundings. You know where you are and where you are going; who you are and what you need to do. Confidence starts with realizing your insecurities and recognizing that these insecurities are YOUR perceptions of yourself – not anyone else's perception of you. Pay close attention to that quiet, little insecure voice of yours whispering to you that you are not good enough or pretty enough to do what you really want to do or look how you want to look. When you hear that voice, and sometimes you have to listen very closely because you are so used to it in the background, just shut it down. Hear it, acknowledge it, and trash it! Inner peace is a wonderful drug that is more effective for many people than medication. It takes lots of practice but you can absolutely control your thoughts and 'self talk'. You'll be amazed at what you can accomplish.

Speaking of accomplishments, they all take time and effort. Great things usually don't just happen. Great accomplishments are a thing of wonder and awe – when someone does something wonderful, we are in awe of them and may even stand there looking at them blankly, mouth open, drooling. Try to hold it together and realize that person has made mistakes along the way. Haven't we all? It is very helpful to look at mistakes as learning opportunities to get better at whatever it is we do. And be thankful – yes be thankful for everything you have because there are so many others that have so much less.

One last tidbit - try to avoid being a perfectionist. According to the Merriam-Webster dictionary, perfectionism is defined as "a disposition to regard anything short of perfection is unacceptable"[1]. This is difficult for most of us when it comes to our face, skin, or body. One little blemish or pimple can turn our world upside down whenever we pass by a mirror or have to speak to someone face to face. Many people wouldn't even notice that zit on your cheek until you point it out so just ignore it - no one cares but you. But all of us probably have some degree of perfectionism in us or the world might be a little more chaotic. The key is to believe that you do not have to be perfect to be loved or that everything has to be perfect for you to accept it. Don't wait for the perfect time for you to begin your project or take that vacation!

Improving your skin or erasing some of the small cruelties of Mother Nature is your right, so go ahead and join "the Club"! According to many happy patients, you will look better and a little fresher, and even feel a little better if you indulge yourself with some Botox, Dysport or fillers or maybe a laser treatment. All you have to do is look at the numbers of non-surgical cosmetic treatments that are done every year. The American Society of Plastic Surgeons (2012)[2] reports over 12 million people have received these treatments, not surgeries, in 2011. That number consistently increases because more people try these treatments when they learn about the aesthetic or beauty benefits they can offer. Cosmetic treatments and procedures tailored to your unique face and personality by a trained practitioner can give you a boost that will make you feel more beautiful and confident.

Confidence shows through your appearance like your favorite camisole under your brand spanking new chiffon blouse. And confidence is essential for feeling your best. It's not thrilling to hear this over and over again but it really is true, even if you're not feeling your most confident self, if you act confident the feeling will follow. Fabulous!

Let's kiss and make-up

Ah yes, make-up. Women are luckier than men because we can wear make-up every single day and camouflage all kinds of things. Men often don't take advantage of the wonders of make-up but women can enhance things like our beautiful eyes, cheeks, and lips. (Men can do it too). Some men look absolutely fabulous in make-up (think Johnny Depp in Pirates) but they typically don't get to run around with lipstick and eyeliner on too often unless they work at the make-up counter at your favorite department store. You don't need to wear a ton. Just enough to give you a little sparkle, and no that doesn't mean glitter.

Way back in the old days, women used all kinds of things to 'enhance' their appearance. Over the centuries women used ash to darken their eyes, berries to stain their lips, and believe it or not, young boys urine to blend freckles[3]. Using make-up is nothing new and we have been using cosmetics for a long time but thankfully we have made some progress!

That being said, lots of people, both men and women wear make-up today. As a matter of fact – everyone on TV and in films must wear make-up or else they would look washed out and sallow. Hmmm, realizing a theme here? Make-up helps you look more alive at work when you've had that one last martini before collapsing on your bed the night before. Make-up when applied correctly, accentuates your fabulousness, doesn't cover it up or mask it. Plus it also camouflages that tiny imperfection you see when you look in the 10x mirror and wonder why you can't look airbrushed in real-life – oh well.

"Make-up can enhance your natural beauty. *The trick is, less is more.* Heavy, thick foundation and powder can accentuate fine lines and wrinkles and make them stand out. For example, use a tinted moisturizer instead of a rich foundation; this will allow the moisturizer to absorb a bit into the skin and not lay on top of it like thicker foundations. For the eyes, stay away from heavy frosted and glitter eye shadows; this ages your appearance.

Stick to neutral tones that will make your eyes pop no matter what color they are. Simplicity is key!" *Jenna Norwood, celebrity make-up artist and medical aesthetician.*

How many times do you leave the house without make-up? Ever? There are countless quotes in magazines from women who refuse to leave the house without "at least lipstick and mascara on". These are the women who always run into someone at the grocery store who looks perfect from her toenails to her headband. Ah, have you ever snuck out of the house just to pick something up – real quick - and ran into someone you wish you wouldn't have run into? If you're running around in sweat pants and no make-up the first thing you want to say is, "oh my gawd, I look awful!" That's a big mistake because you probably look great, maybe even scrubbed clean! One suggested rule to follow is 'never apologize for how you look', because that allows someone else to judge you and dictate how you feel about yourself – forget that! It's about confidence in yourself and allowing you to be you. Make-up is like an accessory that should be worn when you want to snazz things up a bit or look "put together". It does not define who you are. That's taking it a little too far. Make-up not only makes our outside look better but it can make our inside feel better; or instill confidence.

An absolute must for make-up is the practice and talent to be good at application. Try this out; go to the make-up counters at your favorite department store. Scope the place out and look for someone, male or female, whose face you like. (Hint: some of the best make-up artists are men. Think Max Factor, Kevin Aucoin). Don't worry, you don't have to buy a thing, you can take their advice and purchase things at their counter or elsewhere. Look at their skin, color choices, and amount of make-up they use on themselves. Determine if they would help you in your beauty quest by chatting with them first to see if they would be interested in helping you. Then, let the person you choose have a little fun with your face. You might be surprised. Since you never stop learning, try new tips with make-up as part of your beauty process. Remember, as we age our face and make-up needs change so we really should update our routines occasionally.

Despite the need for updating and adjusting make-up routines, there are so many stories about women who have been applying make-up for years and years and are somewhat resistant to having make-up lessons at the make-up counter at their favorite department store. The following is a true story: (WARNING! This may sound familiar)

There once was a woman who was very reluctant to have anyone touch her face and would never entertain the thought of someone putting make-up on her! She's been applying her own makeup for years and is quite happy with herself and how she looks. She does get compliments, you know.

One day she went to her favorite department store and was perusing the makeup

department when all of the sudden, a man about 40 years old leaped out from behind the counter with a huge grin and said "Hi there! I love your eye shadow – it looks fabulous with your eye color!" She immediately noticed HE was wearing a hint of foundation and mascara – yes! Foundation and mascara! She wasn't sure what to make of this situation. He asked if she had ever noticed the section of her eyes that she had been missing with eyeliner. "What do you mean, missing?" she inquired. He handed her a mirror and said, "See? Here" He pointed out the bare area of the upper inside lid that seemed to stand out as a big blank only after he pointed it out to her. "Yes! I see that" she exclaimed. He then showed her a picture of a model in a magazine and showed her exactly what he was talking about. Sure enough, the model's eyes were lined on the inside of her upper lid and looked fantastic! He went on to say that he was working at that particular store for a special event that day as he is usually applying make-up for magazine shoots. He said this is a secret they use to make the model's eyes appear more defined and awake.

After hearing this secret and trusting his expertise, she happily sat in his chair as he applied the liner to her eyes. When he was done, all she could say was "Wow". It made a big difference in her appearance and now that tidbit is part of her daily routine.

The point of this story is that no matter what we already know, we can always learn something new. Life is about learning and exploring and enjoying yourself. Try not to become so set in your ways you can't try anything new or different. It is hard, though. Once you hit 40 (and you'll see what I mean if you're not there already), you seem to get nice and comfortable with the choices you've made and the experiences you've had and don't feel like it's really necessary to do or learn anything new. Well, take a chance and try something you've never tried before; sushi, skydiving, ice-skating or dare I say it, Botox! It's FUN! What have you got to lose?

Dressing? Oh, on the side please

New clothes and shoes…awwww, don't they make you feel good, at least for a while? It's fun to have something new to wear, like you've refurbished yourself for the day. A wonderful costume if you will, maybe that's why Halloween can be so much fun for us adults.

As a kid, it was such a thrill to shop for new school clothes every year, wasn't it? Didn't you love it – picking out things you really liked and spending the day with mom? Growing up, my family didn't have a lot of money but my sister and I always seemed to get at least one pair of Dittos or Jordache jeans and some Wallabies or Vans shoes – magnificent! New duds signified a new beginning, new friends, new teachers, and new chapters to discover. The old clothes saw the inside of a good-will bag or made their way to a garage sale – bye-bye! Off to 9th grade class, looking sharp.

Today most women think shopping still feels great even though now we're the ones paying for everything. At least we get to hang out with our friends. What happened to the good ol' days of whining until we got what we wanted and then having it handed to us at no charge? (Some of us might still do that but that's another story). All we had to do was clean our room or eat our vegetables. We didn't realize how good we had it until our very first credit card bill came and we had completely forgotten what we bought because the bill came 45 days after the purchase. By then, the novelty of our sparkling new purchase had worn off. Shoot! Now we're paying for something that doesn't give us that thrill it once did, a mere month ago.

Although this is nothing new, lots of people have the same nostalgic feelings of new beginnings when buying something new to wear. The key is to really shop for yourself and not base your decisions for purchase on something or someone else. Here are a couple of handy tips for dressing successfully.

TIP #1: Dress for your body and not what's in style – LOVE WHAT YOU BUY!!! Do not succumb to pressure from your friends or sales people – you are the master of your credit card and your style fate. You might have a closet half full of things you do not wear because you do not love them! UGH! If you don't love it at the department store, you will not love it at home. As a matter of fact, have you ever thought they have 'trick' mirrors in the dressing rooms? Like they have some sort of slimming mirror and flattering lighting? Well, imagine, if you buy something in those circumstances with specific lighting and you don't really love it, how do you think you'll feel when you get it home and put it on? You'll likely feel like a moose on the tundra...large, cold and alone. Women have an "intuition" about most things, and clothes are one of them. Go with your gut and do not buy that homely rag!

TIP #2: Avoid too much trend. Trend is just that, a trend. Maybe it's an evil ploy by the designers and magazine editors of the world so they can constantly have a hand in your pocketbook. They are always re-inventing. We are always buying. Have a couple of trendy things that you won't mind setting on fire in about 6 months but stick mainly to the classics unless you have unlimited funding for clothes. How embarrassing to be caught wearing leg warmers in this day and age! Oops – they're back... Well, for a little while anyway.

TIP #3: Lastly, try not to put too much stock in sizes. Your girth is your girth. When you go shopping, depending on the designer of the item, you could be anywhere from a 1 (United States) to a 44 (Italian). No kidding! A common range for a skirt might be 4 to 10 for someone with a 26-inch waist, again depending on the maker of the item. So who cares about size? Weight, well that's another issue.

Some weight tables describe a weight *range* as being healthy or ideal. Depending on your *height* and *frame* the listed weights could range by over 30 lbs. That cannot be very accurate. A very good source used by health care providers is the BMI (body mass index) chart listed on the CDC website that uses the below formula to determine your BMI. This measurement is a better predictor of health and is more specifically categorized to help people achieve or maintain a healthy weight [4]. The categories are:

BMI	Weight Status
Below 18.5	Underweight
18.5 – 24.9	Normal
25.0 – 29.9	Overweight
30.0 and Above	Obese

English Units: BMI = Weight (lb) / (Height (in) x Height (in)) x 703

Example: Someone who is 5'6" (5'6" = 66") and weighs 160 lbs. has a BMI of:

BMI Calculation = 160 / (66 x 66) x 703 = **25.8**.

This person is in the Overweight category.

Following a diet plan appropriate for *you* is the best one for you to stick with and stay healthy. If you need help in meal planning or information on healthy diets, contact a local nutritionist or hospital dietician they are wonderful resources

Diet – the original 4-letter word

Yes, D-I-E-T. Yuck! Diets suck…but we all seem to be on one, like it or not. Some diets are healthy and some are not. Diet is just another name for everything we consume, food-wise. So some of us are on a fast food diet, some of us are on a see-food diet, and some of us are on a plain old diet-diet. Wouldn't it be wonderful to live in a world where we could just eat whatever we want whenever we want to? Oh, the gloriousness of gluttony.

Unfortunately, if we want to stay healthy, we have to take care in what we choose to put into our bodies. Foods that are naturally grown without use of pesticides are ideal – many of these foods are labeled organic. In a perfect world, we should all be eating organic foods, i.e. fruits and vegetables. Meat is a different story. Farm raised, (real farms like out in the country, not "farms" where animals are treated inhumanely and slaughtered by people without regard for animal life) cows, chickens, turkeys are best since they are not raised in filth and fed filth[5]. Additionally, high intake of red meat is associated with colon cancer among other illnesses[6]. Some people claim to be vegetarians, eating fruit and vegetables but then add, "Oh, I only eat chicken and fish". Last we checked chicken and fish were not fruit or vegetables.

Exercise

Oh yes we all love to exercise, don't we? Don't we all look forward to running miles and miles on a treadmill or reluctantly hoisting our bodies up onto an elliptical machine? How about lifting weights, mountain bike riding, and spin class – oooooh what fun! Wait a minute, someone mentioned Zumba class and that it is actually fun, or so they say. The truth is one of the reasons people exercise is because of the feeling they get during and especially afterwards, they feel great. Studies have shown over and over that exercise releases chemicals in the brain that trigger and excite our happy place and make us feel good.[7] Heard of runner's high? Well, it's real but it can take quite a bit of time to get that high, (did you read that right?). But, and that's a big butt, it seems to be worth the effort because millions and millions of people exercise every day.

Can you think of a day you drove hurriedly by someone jogging, walking the dog, or bike riding when you were on your way to work? Boy, I'll bet you were glad you weren't out there sweating and huffing and puffing – yuck! You were probably not thinking…'gee I wish that was me' but you might feel a twinge of guilt and quietly wish to yourself that you had gotten up a little earlier and engaged in some kind of exercise. Ah, the joy of being done with a workout. Not only do people love the good feeling they get from exercise but also the burning of extra calories. This helps us feel better about ourselves (as long as we don't eat everything in sight after we're finally off the treadmill).

Speaking of feeling better, try not to listen too much to those blessed super models and celebrities who are so thin they have to shop in the children's section because they "just can't gain weight" or don't have any diet plan because "I just eat whatever I want". Diets of cigarettes and sodas aren't the best thing for your health or your body, not to mention your skin. Truthfully, most people have to invest blood, sweat, and tears to look halfway decent in a tunic, much less a nail-biting swimsuit. Yes, unfortunately, we all should exercise and it's a reality that exercise has many benefits, so try to do it sometime. You'll thank "YOU" for it.

Products

HEADLINE NEWS! Miracle of miracles! All of the answers to all of your problems are in this little jar, tube, or packet. Yes! Buy this cream and your skin will be like a 2-month old baby's skin! No more wrinkles, no more lines! This one has the extract from a Bumble Bee's antennae found deep in the forest under the only blossom tree with pink leaves in the Fairytale district of Make Believe Isle! This rare, miraculous cream can be yours for only $300 a ¼ ounce – hooray!

Well, the real secret is to get products that really work and *use* them. You can't expect one facial to give you glowing skin for months, can you? You go to the dentist and get your teeth cleaned but you certainly brush your teeth at home, don't you? You need to find products that suit your skin and give you the results you're looking for but the real deal is you have to *use* those products. So many women say "oh yes, I have that product" but it's sitting in their cabinet ever so lonely since it never comes out to play, uh, work. Others say "Oh yeah, I tried that one too but it didn't work" but sometimes time is the culprit. We all want everything so quickly, that instant gratification, and when a product takes longer than 2 days to see results, we throw in the towel. Even prescription products can take a while before you see results. Patience my dear, patience. More on skin care products in the next chapter.

Botox, Dysport, Fillers – oh my!

Botox and Dysport, along with dermal fillers such as Restylane, Perlane, and Juvederm have a long track record of being safe and effective. Millions of men and women have these treatments every year and every year those numbers grow, seemingly regardless of the economy. These are the treatments that turn back the hands of time and make you wonder, "How does she look so good?" These treatments offer real alternatives to the surgical procedures that were once required to achieve improvements in appearance. Now with a few tiny injections and a bit of strategically placed volume with dermal fillers, we can wipe some of our lines and folds away for a fraction of what a surgical procedure might cost.

Many women who have not tried Botox are fearful for one reason or another. Most commonly, it's because they think the "toxin" or "poison" will travel through their bodies and render them paralyzed or dysfunctional. The truth is Botox and Dysport are highly purified proteins derived from the botulinum toxin molecule. Basically, the cosmetic form of Botox and Dysport work by blocking the nerve impulse when a molecule, from our own bodies, acetycholine (pronounced ah-seat-il-koe-leen), tries to activate muscle movement.[8] After about 3-4 months, the molecules have dissolved and your skin returns to baseline and you have full muscle movement again. It doesn't matter if you're the Queen of England, the effect of Botox and Dysport lasts 3-4 months, that's about it. However, there are a small amount of patients who say their Botox effects last 6 – 8 months but that is a rarity and isn't the case with most people. And some have experienced that ongoing treatments can lessen the need to go in as often.

One of the reasons Botox is so effective and in such high demand is because it smooth's the lines that make us appear stressed or angry. Years and years of squinting and frowning can take a toll on our face. Remember all those years of squinting and frowning might not be smoothed away after just one treatment either. Depending on the depth of your lines and bulk of your muscles, it may take several treatments to get a really smooth look and then, of course, you'll need to maintain it with subsequent treatments. Don't worry though, if the lines between your brows are super deep and you can "feel" the "dents", you may be a candidate for Botox or Dysport and then a tiny bit of a filler to plump up the area. No, you won't look like Frankenstein with a lovely, bossy, voluptuous forehead. You'll look nice and smooth. You and your friends won't believe what a difference "smoothing out" does for this little area on our face. People won't think you're mad all the time...

Lights, Camera, Action!

Ah the beauty of light. Light is miraculous. Light does so many things; makes things grow, lets us see what the hell we're doing, and (according to some books and movies), guides us where to go when we die. But more importantly, it gets rid of unwanted hair, reverses sun damage, lightens pigments, lessens unsightly vessels, evens out our skin tone, reduces wrinkles, and stimulates collagen growth – wow, now you're talking! The types of light that does these wonderful things are lasers and intense pulsed light (IPL). There are many different types of devices out there that will help you get your skin into shape and certain types can even rid you of most of your unwanted hair. These treatments will be discussed in detail in Chapters 4 and 7 but it is very important you find an experienced and highly trained practitioner because serious adverse reactions can occur. Lasers – hello!

You cutey, you

Above all, don't feel like you have to conform to society's standard of beauty – conform to your own standards. You're reading this book because you probably want to learn something about what real women do to become and stay as beautiful as they can. If you don't like applying make-up, try to get over it. A little can do wonders.

Try new things; see if you like microdermabrasion or Botox or Restylane or other things. Keep an open mind and discover what millions of others have discovered. Let's let the cat out of the bag and give away the secrets to beauty!

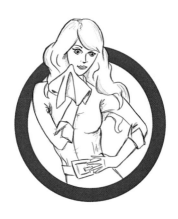

Chapter 2

SKIN CARE

Oh glorious skin!

Our skin is such a wonderful organ, constantly changing, protecting our bodies, and regulating our temperature. It is truly amazing and we should treat it with care and respect.

Let's briefly review some of the skin's fascinating structures and functions. Don't worry, there won't be a lot of nerdy science stuff here but you should know the basics if you want to take a more active part in caring for and protecting your largest organ.

Let's start with the *epidermis*. Yes we've all heard that joke in second grade "hey, your epidermis is showing!" and then we laugh as our unsuspecting friend positions his hands over his crotch. Well, the reality is, your epidermis IS showing. It's the top layer of your skin. It is composed of 4 distinct layers made up of different cell types that do different things.

Basically, the epidermis is our protective layer that is constantly undergoing renewal. This is the area where the brown spots, fine lines and other effects of aging and sun damage are apparent. Skin cells shed approximately every 21-28 days depending on your age. Younger people tend to shed skin cells every 21 days or so[1]. This layer also provides mechanical protection to the underlying skin cells and in addition, acts as a barrier to help prevent water loss and invasion of foreign substances. Pretty impressive, huh?

The next layer is the *dermis*. This layer houses the sweat glands, hair follicles, and oil (sebaceous) glands as well as nerve endings and blood vessels. There are three kinds of sweat glands; one regulates heat (eccrine), the other two, scent release (apocrine) and (apoeccrine). The eccrine sweat glands are most plentiful in the feet and least plentiful on the back. The apocrine and apoeccrine sweat glands are confined mainly to the underarms and perineum[2] (taint). Explains a lot, doesn't it? Lastly, the apoeccrine sweat glands have been implicated in what is called hyperhidrosis, or abnormally increased rates of perspiration[3]. If you already know what this is, you probably suffer from it. This condition is fairly common and causes embarrassment to many people, especially women and teenagers. Sweaty underarms and palms that are not controlled by the usual antiperspirants are annoying and cause distress. Our magical, secret weapon

Botox works wonders for this condition - way to go vitamin B!

Hair follicles are another component of the dermis. We are born with all of the approximately 5 million hair follicles we will ever have - none are added after we are born[4]. They do however become active at different times of life, think puberty and menopause, and also respond to different medications. The hair shaft itself contains cells called melanosomes (cells that are responsible for our hair color). Loss of these cells as we age causes the hair to become gray[5]. Lasers used for hair removal target the melanosomes in the hair and alter or destroy the hair follicle so it cannot produce hair. More of this will be discussed in the chapter on lasers but you get the idea. So if you've waited too long to get those pesky chin hairs treated by a laser and now they are gray, you can get electrolysis and make those hairs disappear with a hot needle. Fun.

An additional feature of the skin and hair follicle is the sebaceous (oil) gland. These glands are most abundant on the face and scalp and produce sebum that acts as a lubricant[6]. Oil on our face and hair is actually good for the skin and helps keep it moist and, you guessed it, youthful.

Believe it or not, fingernails and toenails are a component of the skin. The nails provide protection to the fingertips and toes, help us grab things, and are used for scratching that itch. The nails grow approximately 0.5mm to 1.2mm per day and fingernails grow faster than toenails. The nails grow like hair, from the base but they do not have a resting phase like hair does – nails keep on growing. Fingernails and toenails are made of the superficial type of skin cells, the stratum corneum, (the dead, upper most cells on our skin) but the nails include hard keratin[7]. These cells are already dead and have no sensation so you can painlessly clip and cut them. You can also dress them up for parties.

Nerves, blood vessels and specialized cells that are associated with allergic response, inflammation, and immunity are also contained in the skin. There are specialized cells located within the skin that send signals and messages to other cells to respond in case of allergens or other irritants. These in turn cause the reactions, swellings, pain, itching, and redness that can happen when the skin comes in contact with poison ivy or a chemical it doesn't like[8]. It really is a magnificent organ, always trying to protect us.

The last layer of the skin discussed here will be the subcutaneous fat layer. We are born with lots of fat cells to keep us warm. The bummer is that the cells themselves have unlimited capacity to grow. Each cell can balloon up and increase our girth quite easily, as many of us have observed. The subcutaneous fat acts as a storage house for energy and provides our bodies with buoyancy in water[9]. So, next time you see someone who is overweight, you can just think of them as, buoyant. It's more polite.

Sun exposure; we love it, we hate it

Prolonged (over 30 minutes unprotected or burning) sun exposure is one of the worst things you can do to yourself and your skin, especially if you are fair or light skinned. Your poor skin is trying to protect you by creating dark spots that will help absorb more of the sun's harmful UVA and UVB rays. That's why the skin gets tan and creates freckles and brown patches; darker skin absorbs the damaging cancer and wrinkle causing rays. And sunburn is the worst! Sunburnt cells actually undergo programmed cell death as a result of irreparable DNA damage from the UV radiation. Isn't that sad? By sun burning your skin, even once, you're killing your beautiful little skin cells one at a time. These changes in the DNA of the skin cells can lead to several different kinds of skin cancer including melanoma, which is deadly.

Now, take a look at your chest, do you see a bunch of crinkly, old-looking skin? Be honest. Sometimes your skin can't keep up with all of the radiation from the sun and so it gives up and then slowly the fibers that help keep our skin taut and youthful looking, start breaking up. Contrary to popular belief, breaking up is not hard to do.

The fibers that keep our skin youthful are *collagen* and *elastin*: These structures lie a bit deeper in the skin but eventually succumb to the damage caused by sun exposure because the harmful rays from the sun penetrate to their level[10]. The poor things just become weak and frail and eventually break down allowing your skin to sag and wrinkle. Yes, it takes a while, sometimes years for these signs of damage to start showing up, but boy our mirrors have no problem telling us when it's too late.

Kids nowadays are pretty lucky because they have moms who are conscious about their own skin as well as their child's skin. Moms are now starting to look in the mirror and see these little lines and wrinkles making their debut; then they snatch the sunscreen and drown their child with it.

Ah, but too little too late for us in our 30's, 40's and 50's. We didn't know better. We used aluminum shields to direct the sun's rays right onto our faces and chest and even used baby oil with a hint of iodine in it so we had instant color – yippee! One summer day when I was 13, I ran out of my beloved baby oil and in sheer desperation, I used Vaseline, (yes the gooey petroleum jelly), to really bake in the sun. What a mess. It took 3 showers to get the shiny, sun damage inducing jelly, off my skin. I got the worst ever burn and was red for days. (Back in those days, boys really liked lobsters).

Anyway, the point is, that teenagers, parents, and most other people now know that baking in the sun is not healthy for your skin, especially if you would like to look 30 when you're 40, or 30-ish when you're 50. Healthy skin is important, not just for looks, but for your protection. When skin gets crinkly, small abrasions and cracks allow bacteria, chemicals, and other toxins into the skin and this can cause infection and further skin breakdown. The following are some ideas about skin care and sunscreens. Not to be too serious, but here are some important facts everyone should know:

Hydrate

It's important to drink plenty of water. Sixty-four ounces of water per day is recommended for the average, healthy person for overall health and skin care. Water helps carry nutrients into the cells and assists in waste and toxin removal from the body. Without enough water flowing through the body, these toxins can build up and escape through the skin, and may contribute to acne. Some experts believe drinking water keeps the skin plumper and more youthful looking. Without water, dehydration sets in causing the skin to appear dry and can also contribute to other health problems such as electrolyte imbalances.

Sun Protection – The sun is not always our friend

First, let's figure out what "Skin Type" you are. Don't worry; this will just take a second. Look at the chart and see which category your skin is associated with. This is a guide, based on what happens to your un-tanned skin, in spring, after the first 60 minutes of sun exposure[11]. See chart on next page.

Fitzpatrick Skin Type: Sun History:

I (lightest, white)	Always burns easily, never tans, extremely sun-sensitive skin
II (light, white)	Usually burns easily, tans minimally, very sun-sensitive skin
III (white – olive)	Sometimes burns, gradually tans to light brown, sun sensitive skin
IV (light brown)	Burns minimally, tans to moderate brown, minimally sun-sensitive
V (brown)	Rarely burns, tans well
VI (dark brown, black)	Never burns, tans deeply

Don't freak out if you fall between two categories. For safety sake, regarding sun exposure, always go the next level *up*. For example if you sometimes burn (type III) but have very sun sensitive skin (type II), pick skin type II because you will use more sun protection. Now, brace yourself – this next part is confusing.

The *opposite* goes for laser or IPL treatments; higher or darker skin types are treated *less* aggressively than lighter skin types because darker skin types absorb more IPL and laser light energy with MORE side effects, like burns. The reason for this is because people with darker skin types have more melanin in their skin. These cells absorb more light and transform it into more intense heat and this can lead to burning of the skin. So, your experienced practitioner will use expert clinical judgment and use an energy level that is safe for you. More on IPL will be forthcoming in chapter 4. Regardless of your skin type, you need to wear a broad-spectrum (protection from both UVA and UVB rays) water-resistant sunscreen, year round!

Sunscreen is crucial in protecting our skin from damage from the sun's rays. There are two kinds of rays, ultraviolet A (UVA) and ultraviolet B (UVB). Alarmingly, UVA passes through window glass and causes most of the aging and wrinkles whereas UVB radiation does not pass through glass but is responsible for burns and long term effects such as skin cancer[12]. A good way to remember these rays is UVA – "A" for aging and UVB – "B" for burning. Although both will eventually cause aging, wrinkles, and cancer so you need protection from both and not just in summer!

So you see, when the indoor tanning salon staff naively tell you they have "controlled environments" or use only "safe" UVA or UVB rays in their beds, you will now know that indoor tanning is not safe or healthy. As a matter of fact, tanning beds and sun lamps are known cancer-causing agents[13]. You can't really blame these cute, young, thin, tan girls who work in tanning salons.

They are just like we were yet they have fast-acting tanning beds and we had the beach, the pool and the park.

Sunscreens that offer protection from both kinds of rays are called "broad spectrum". Broad-spectrum protection is highly recommended by health care clinicians and skin care specialists. These sunscreens should be used all year long – even on cloudy days because the sun's damaging rays can penetrate through clouds. Over and over again, people say "but I don't lay in the sun!" Yet, they are in the office for crinkly, saggy skin solutions to the *damage caused by the sun*. Further conversation with these ladies reveals most of these types of patients (you?) are very active. Either playing tennis, running or gardening, but none-the-less, outside, and most times "just in the morning".

Sadly, facts are facts and the fact is these early morning outside activities include sun exposure. Yes, the strongest radiation from the sun is between the hours of 10:00 AM and 2:00 PM however, there are plenty of other damaging rays *all day long.*

Another frequent complaint from patients with sun-damaged skin is, "But I wear sunscreen and I'm still getting color!" Yes, this can be very frustrating. They are diligent about putting sunscreen on in the morning before they go out to the beach or shopping but it is very difficult to remember to re-apply when you're on your third margarita. Plus, who wants to put on more of that gooier sunscreen, especially when it's 90 or 100 degrees outside, much less put it on over makeup (if you're wearing any). There are several options in powder

36

sunscreens also available and they work great for us who wear make-up at the beach or river because we can apply the powder right over our make-up or other sunscreens! Yee-haw!

Oh no, here comes another bothersome fact – you must wear *and re-apply* sunscreens. Even more distressing is there are reports stating that not only sun exposure causes some of the brown pigments but heat from the sun stimulates this phenomenon as well. Not only that, you need to use sunscreens that have certain ingredients that act as sunscreens for the sunscreens. Oh jeez...WHAT?!

Sunscreens that contain avobenzone, Mexoryl (UVA) and octocrylene (UVB) are effective broad-spectrum applications. Certain combinations provide increased sunscreen stability because the sun's rays break down plain old sunscreen[14]. Other popular and effective sunscreens contain titanium dioxide and zinc oxide, however some leave a white residue on the skin that is noticeable and, unless you want to look like a polar bear, this is not the best look. There is a plethora of over-the-counter sunscreens and others that are useful and widely available in medical spas, dermatology offices, drug stores, and department stores.

Broad Spectrum UV Ingredients

Mexoryl

Avobenzone	Octyl salicylate
Cinoxate	Oxybenzone
Ecamsule	Sulisobenzone
Menthyl anthranilate	Titanium dioxide
Octyl methoxycinnamate	Zinc oxide

**The FDA requires that all sunscreens be stable and remain at their original strength for at least 3 years – unless indicated by an expiration date[15].

Because the amount of sun exposure varies significantly from person to person and there are many factors to consider, re-application is essential for everyone. When evaluating sunburn protection factor (SPF), it is best to take into consideration the amount of sun exposure you will receive, time of day, geographical location, and weather conditions. The recommended SPF is 30 to 50 and even higher, however, the new Food and Drug Administration (FDA) rulings state the highest rating will be 50+ and the terms "sun-block, sweat-proof, and water-proof" will no longer be allowed[16]. The SPF of 30 provides about 97% protection when it is applied correctly.

A novel new sunscreen out on the market is an internal one – that's right, you drink a capful about an hour prior to sun exposure! It's called Harmonized Water

– UV protection and it claims to offer sun protection of "30 times more than normal" by neutralizing UV rays and isolating the frequencies of the rays through our skin. This product needs to be taken again in 3 hours if you are out in the sun for extended periods. One advantage to this internal sunscreen is you won't feel like you're wearing sticky sunscreen but a disadvantage may be that it is not as effective as traditional sunscreens or may not be effective at all. The science is still evolving.

Remember UVA = Aging, UVB = Burning. Both lead to cancer and ugly skin. For those of us that have enjoyed or still enjoy basking in sunny days and catching those sunny rays, read on for ways to help your skin look better.

Select active ingredients, for real results!
Skin lighteners and blenders

Topical skin preparations that include hydroquinone, kojic acid, or Retin-A and its derivatives, improve skin appearance by lightening darker pigments and helping to prevent the activity of cells that produce freckling or hyperpigmentation. Sun exposure can result in unsightly brown spots or freckles whereas another condition, melasma, has several suggested causes including estrogen, heat, along with sun exposure. Melasma is a common, acquired disorder that usually presents with symmetric hyper-pigmented or brown patches on the face particularly in pregnancy[17]. Multiple laser modalities have been used for melasma, but treatment results are highly variable and recurrence after treatment is common. Worsening of hyperpigmentation or mottled hypopigmentation may also occur as a result of laser therapy so it is not the first choice in treating this condition. Topical preparations are best.

Mechanism of Action (Hydroquinone)

For you brainiacs: Hydroquinone works by producing reversible depigmentation of the skin by suppressing the melanocyte metabolic processes, in particular the inhibition of the enzymatic oxidation of tyrosine to DOPA (3,4-dihydroxyphenylalanine); sun exposure reverses this effect and will cause re-pigmentation[18]. Say that three times fast.

There are several popular prescription skin lightening products and regimens containing hydroquinone that work over several months to blend the pigments of the skin to make it look more even-toned and radiant. Most people get remarkable results, however, some regimens have multiple steps and products that can be cumbersome and difficult for some people to use, especially if their current skin care regimen includes only one or two steps. Many people only use a cleanser and moisturizer and think this is sufficient. Sadly, it isn't, especially if you have any pigment concerns. The problem with more complex regimens is people want instant results (including us!), and they don't want to have to work at it (think exercise). There are a few other prescription products available containing Retin-A derivatives and hydroquinone that are manufactured as a single product and these combination products can make the whole skin care process easier.

Kojic Acid

Kojic acid has the same effect on the skin as hydroquinone and is found in many skin care products. Kojic acid is derived from the Aspergillus oryzae fungus and is an effective alternative to hydroquinone. Kojic acid has been shown to be equally as effective as hydroquinone although it has been reported to be slightly more irritating and can cause an increase in slight peeling. An observation by some patients is the hydroquinone takes on a brownish tinge when it begins to oxidize where the kojic acid does not - some care, some don't[19].

Retin-A

Retin-A or retinoids is a wonderful tool to have in your skin care arsenal. Retin – A is a vitamin A derivative and if you use it with hydroquinone you should notice substantial and marvelous skin lightening and blending results, although it does take some time. To be honest, up to several months. Yes, yes, we all want instant results but unfortunately, more youthful, blended skin can take a while. Think about it, your poor skin took years of abuse and yet always remained by your side, well your outside. There it was, absorbing all that radiation from the sun and you just went on your merry way like nothing was happening. Ignoring your skin, tanning your skin, or (gasp!) *burning* your skin. So sad, sniff, sniff. Ah, but now the time has come. You've taken a close look at your skin and decided to do something about those brown spots and that worn out collagen. And, you've decided you want everything all better right now! Well, it's all over except the crying.

Mechanism of Action (Retinoids)

Keratinocytes (those dead skin cells that need to shed off the body) in the sebaceous follicle (the pore where the hair grows out) become less sticky which allows for easy removal and sloughing. It also inhibits microcomedone formation (small black heads) and eliminates lesions already present[20].

In a nutshell, retinoids help the skin cells that would normally slough off do just that, slough off. Problems happen when those cells get stuck in the oil glands and hair follicles, those problems being rough skin and acne. We think scientists were studying the effects of retinoids on patients with acne and noticed their skin looked fabulously smooth and less wrinkled. "Boy", they must have thought that teenagers and women will, "gobble this stuff up!" Numma-num…

Retin – A: Warnings/Precautions

Some concerns related to adverse effects:

• *Photosensitivity*: Use of retinoid products is associated with increased susceptibility/sensitivity to UV light and can cause redness and irritation; avoid sunlamps or excessive sunlight exposure. Daily sunscreen use and other protective measures are highly recommended, duh.

• *Skin irritation*: Use of these products can increase skin sensitivity to weather extremes of wind or cold. Also, additional topical medications like medicated or abrasive cleansers, or cosmetics with a strong drying effect should be used with caution due to possible increased skin irritation[21].

On a side note: we women purchase so many products with the "hope" that it will work on our wrinkles, red blotches, brown blotches, scars, fat, cellulite, stretch marks, whatever. The cosmetic and beauty cream industry is a multi-billion dollar market yet if these "amazing" wrinkle creams really worked, wouldn't it make huge headlines? Wouldn't one or two companies wipe out most of the others? Wouldn't we all have empty jars of the stuff all over our bathrooms and vanities? Why yes...but look around your medicine cabinet – go ahead, I'll wait. What did you see? Bet you saw so many jars, tubes, canisters, and bottles more than half full of the newest and latest "miracle" cream or potion it made you wonder what kind of car you could've bought with all the money you spent on those products.

Isn't it frustrating? But if something really worked, you use it up and buy more. Think toilet paper. What happens when products really work? We use them, run out of them and buy more of them. We don't buy different products and not the newest or latest "miracle". Yes tons of creams provide moisture but it's the active ingredients that really blend the skin tone, stimulate collagen growth or improve fine lines and many, if not all, of these are prescription products.

The reason these products are prescription is because the Food and Drug Administration (FDA) has deemed them 'drugs'. Drugs are defined by the FDA as "articles intended for use in the diagnosis, cure, mitigation, treatment, or prevention of disease in man or other animals; and (C) articles (other than food) intended to affect the structure or any function of the body of man or other animals"[22]. Subsequently, cosmetics are defined by the FDA as their intended use, as "articles intended to be rubbed, poured, sprinkled, or sprayed on, introduced into, or otherwise applied to the human body...for cleansing, beautifying, promoting attractiveness, or altering the appearance"[23]. Among the products included in this definition are skin moisturizers, perfumes, lipsticks, fingernail polishes, eye and facial makeup preparations, shampoos, permanent waves, hair colors, toothpastes, and deodorants, as well as any material intended for use as a component of a cosmetic product[24]. Additionally, there is a commonly used term "cosmeceutical" but the FDA does not recognize this term under the law. However, there are products that are both drug and cosmetic such as certain make-ups that claim to have sun protection attributes. These products must comply with both drug and cosmetic regulations.

So you see, our regulatory agencies provide clear definitions of what drugs vs. cosmetics are supposed to do. This is a little refreshing because the claims, products, and treatments are so confusing – there are so many!

Antioxidants

Basically, antioxidants protect the skin and body from tiny monsters called free radicals. According to scientists, free radicals are unstable molecules that roam around in your body and skin and steal parts of your healthy molecules called *electrons*. (Let's not dive too deeply into chemistry here but it's nice to understand what is going on in your body and skin). Once these free radicals have collected an electron from a healthy molecule, they cause all kinds of hell; accelerate aging, accumulate toxins and pigments, and trigger changes in the chromosomes, among other things, in your precious skin and body[24]. Does this sound like sun exposure effects? Yes? Wear your sunscreen! By the way, cigarette smoking does the same thing – we know you don't smoke so we don't need to lecture you. Only numbskulls smoke and you're reading this book so you're obviously not a numbskull.

These little free-radical devils are what scientists believe cause aging so this is where good health and good skin care come in. Antioxidants are our defense to these little freaks of nature. There's a good amount of research that shows certain antioxidants in combination with each other provide the most effective defense and repair to the damage caused by free-radials[26]. Antioxidant ingredients like Vitamin C and Vitamin E are also beneficial to skin appearance, not just its health.

Over-the-counter products are too numerous to mention by name but look for ingredients such as vitamins A, E and C, and alpha-hydroxy acids (AHA). Other fabulous ingredients are resveratrol, coffeeberry extract, caffeine, alpha-lipoic acid (ALA), green tea extracts, and alpha-hydroxy acid (see table). These ingredients help protect collagen and prevent cell breakdown in the skin that lead to facial lines and chest, hands, and neck lines too.

Vitamins C and E

Vitamins C (ascorbic acid) and E work synergistically and also have a remarkable ability to penetrate into the skin from topical application. Vitamin C protects and rejuvenates skin, can lighten pigments, and also plays a significant role in collagen synthesis. Unfortunately, our bodies cannot make vitamin C so we need to get it from outside sources, food and topical application.

On the other hand, our sebaceous (oil) glands produce vitamin E, or tocopherol, and provide some defense against environmental stressors like sun exposure and smoking. Topical application of products containing vitamin E is important because if our skin production of vitamin E doesn't keep up with vitamin E depletion from the environment, we lose the protection and here come the wrinkles and brown spots[27].

Other Fabulous Ingredients

Resveratrol – This is produced in the skin of wine grapes. Currently being studied, preliminary findings have shown this powerful anti-oxidant is more potent and absorbed better than current antioxidant formulations[28].

Coffeeberry extract – Coffeeberry has a ton of polyphenols (antioxidants). Topical products that include coffeeberry extract are regarded as safe. Although no conclusive clinical studies assessing topical preparations containing coffeeberry extract have been performed, demonstrating their efficacy in photo-aging and skin cancer prevention, polyphenols in general are known to have a strong antioxidant effect[29,30].

Caffeine – In some studies, topically applied products containing caffeine have shown to have anti-cancer effects, decrease skin roughness and tiny wrinkles. Also may help repair sun damaged skin[31]. Great for inflammation too!

Alpha-lipoic acid (ALA) - This is considered a 'universal' anti-oxidant because it is soluble in both water and fat. It's absorbed well into the skin and can prevent damaging free radicals from doing their destruction. Studies have shown it works wonderfully with Vit. C and E enhancing their effectiveness. In one study, ALA diminished fine lines and brown spots[32,33].

Azelaic acid – Has been shown to be effective for melasma (brown patches of skin on the face), rosacea (redness on the face), and even acne[34].

Green tea extracts (catechins) – This is associated with the most scientific evidence to back up its use in dermatology. It has been found to be an excellent anti-inflammatory, anti-cancer and anti-aging. Make sure you look for products that have about 80-90% polyphenol content for effectiveness since most products contain much less than this[35,36].

Resorcinol – The primary indications for resorcinol are melasma, acne, hyperpigmentation, sun-damaged skin, and freckles[37]. Usually used as a peel.

Alpha-hydroxy (AHA) and beta-hydroxy acids (BHA)- These acids exfoliate the skin leading to smoother *looking, fresher skin. They also increase dermal thickness which aides in the appearance of fine lines[38]. These are very popular ingredients in peels and are also available in take-home products.*

Coenzyme Q10 (CoQ10) - This is a substance that is found naturally in almost every cell in the body; helps convert food into energy, and is a powerful antioxidant. Antioxidants neutralize those free radicals that contribute to the aging process (remember?). Primary dietary sources of CoQ10 include oily fish (such as salmon and tuna), organ meats (such as liver), and whole grains. Most people get enough CoQ10 through a balanced diet, but some people may need supplements if they have certain health conditions[39,40].

Skin Care on a Budget

Many of us don't have the counter space or the money to spend a lot on our basic skin care routine, so here are some tips to help get us through our daily regimens. By the way, this is not just for your face. Following at least some or all of these tips, will help keep your skin as healthy as possible, and looking good too!

TIP #1: Use sunscreen every day. Yes 365 days a year. How many days you ask? The answer is...**365**. That's right, you're reading this correctly. 365 days a year.

TIP #2: Apply your moisturizer as soon as you get out of the tub or shower. Please dry off first – ew. Then immediately put on your moisturizer because this provides an instant layer that locks in moisture.

TIP #3: Vaseline, Aquafor, or petroleum jelly. Yep, that thick greasy stuff works great on feet, elbows, lips and for you athletes, helps with chafing during exercise.

TIP #4: Only use one or two skin care product lines at a time or you're going to be spending a ton of money on products that are likely too similar to make a difference.

TIP #5: Use some kind of product every 12 hours. A cleanser, toner, sunscreen, moisturizer, anything, but you need to do something. Ok?

TIP #6: Avoid too much fragrance in your skin care products, as some tend to lead to skin problems like rashes or sensitivity. Yes, this includes those real expensive products. Paying more does not necessarily mean you're getting a more effective product.

(➔FYI – glycolic acid decreases the stratum corneum barrier function and accelerates the turnover of the skin[41]. This is a good thing because your new, fresh skin is healthier. You can find many products both over the counter and at your clinician's office that contain this ingredient, including some professional peels).

Sleep

Sleep is glorious and we all need it. Some recent studies have found adequate sleep (7 – 8 hours a night) prevents diseases like diabetes and obesity. Others have shown that sleep deprivation of 72 or even 96 hours can lead to temporary psychosis and yet other studies have shown being awake for more than 24 hours straight demonstrated impairment to levels of being drunk![42] No one really knows why we need to sleep but the latest recommendation is about 8 hours each night. Sleep helps our skin somehow and theoretically helps with rejuvenation and repair. Have you ever noticed your skin doesn't look as fresh when you haven't had a good night's sleep? Now go to bed, it's been a long day.

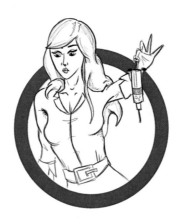

Chapter 3

OVERVIEW OF TREATMENT OPTIONS FOR NEEDLE PHOBICS

Needles? No Thanks!

Ok, as shocking as this might be, not everyone wants Botox. What?! Yes, it's true and for those people, there are several options that help keep your skin in tip-top shape. Keep in mind none of these treatments will give as dramatic a result as say, a laser treatment or IPL, but the results are very noticeable if you maintain a regular schedule of treatments. The treatments we will look at in this chapter are microdermabrasion, chemical peels, and an eyelash treatment. Let's talk about the basic microdermabrasion first.

Microdermabrasion

Microdermabrasion is a non-invasive procedure that removes surface debris and old skin cells from the top layers of your skin. You can get these treatments on your face, neck, chest, hands, arms, almost anywhere on your body where you would like smoother, softer skin. Some areas of the body, such as the vulva (or va-jay-jay), or scalp (unless you have no hair), among other areas, are not appropriate areas for microdermabrasions because it can cause damage to this delicate skin.

Theoretically, microdermabrasion treatments allow serums and other skin care products to more effectively absorb into the skin since it removes the top, rough layer and cleans off other debris. The physical effects of the microdermabrasion actually stimulate new collagen growth by the removal of the outer, dry layer of skin. There is no down time and usually no pain with these treatments. So there isn't a need for topical anesthetic[1]. You can immediately see all of those disgusting dead skin cells trapped in the sponge of the microdermabrasion wand. Yes, the device has a wand, (it's a magical treatment). The effects of the microdermabrasion last about 21 to 28 days depending on the speed of your skin cell turn over. If you are regular about getting these treatments, you can notice improvements in the texture, pigments, clarity, pore appearance, and fine lines[2].

Microdermabrasion is sometimes confused with dermabrasion. Dermabrasion is a surgical procedure performed by a plastic surgeon or dermatologist where the outer most layer of skin is scraped away using a wire brush or a burr containing diamond particles attached to a motorized device[3].

Next, let's learn about peels.

Chemical Peels

Light chemical peels

If you have uneven pigment from sun damage, dryness, acne or fine wrinkling, a light chemical peel might be the right choice for you. This type of peel removes the superficial, outer layer of skin (epidermis) in a light exfoliation and results in a healthier glow. You'll notice even more difference if you have regular peels. The peel chemical is absorbed into the skin and irritates the skin cells so they loosen and eventually peel away. What is revealed is your new, healthy skin from underneath that old yucky layer. Usually, a combination of alpha-hydroxy acids and beta hydroxy acids, such as glycolic acid, lactic acid, salicylic acid and maleic acid are used for these types of peels. All of these chemicals are the mildest choices and you can repeat these treatments weekly for up to six weeks to achieve your desired results[4].

Here's How It Works:

- Your face will be cleansed

- The chemical solution is brushed onto your skin and left on for up to 10 minutes.

- You may feel some mild stinging or tingling

- The solution is then washed off and some types of peels are neutralized with water or a different solution.

- It is recommended to return once a month to maintain your vibrant new look.

Medium chemical peel

If you are one of the many people who suffer with acne scars, more than just fine wrinkles and uneven skin color, you may want to consider a medium chemical peel. The chemicals used for this type of peel will remove skin cells from both the outer layer of skin (epidermis) and upper part of your middle layer of skin (dermis). Trichloroacetic acid (TCA) is sometimes used in combination with glycolic acid and is used at different percentages to achieve desired results. Another popular combination is the Jessner peel that uses a combination of resveratrol, resorcinol, L-lactic acid, salicylic acid and sometimes fruit acids are added as well[5].

Here's How It Works:

- Your face will be cleansed

- The chemical solution is brushed onto your skin and left for just a few minutes.

- You may feel some burning or stinging

- The treated area may turn a whitish grey color

- The chemicals are neutralized if needed

- Your skin may turn red or brown in the days just after the peel.

Recovery varies and can take up to 3-4 weeks for your skin to be back to normal. You may repeat medium chemical peels every 3 to 12 months to maintain your glowing new skin.

Deep chemical peel

The deep chemical peels are used but many practices prefer to use a laser to better control depth. Regardless, here are the aspects of a deep chemical peel.

If you have deeper facial wrinkles, moderately sun damaged skin, scars, or pre-cancerous growths, deep facial chemical peels might be the best choice for you. A physician, *not* an aesthetician, will use the strongest chemical called phenol to penetrate down to the lower dermal layer of your skin[6]. Since this type of peel causes significant discomfort, a local anesthetic and a sedative would likely be used... nitey-night.

Here's How It Works:

- A deep chemical peel usually involves some sort of pretreatment for a few weeks that will prepare your skin for the peel. Pre-treatment can include the use of Retin A – as described previously, a prescription medication that's derived from vitamin A that thins the skin's top layer and allows the peel to travel deeper into the skin.

- You will be given a sedative to relax along with a local anesthetic to numb your face

- Your face will be cleansed

- Phenol is brushed onto the area and is usually left on from 30 minutes but up to two hours. The chemical is neutralized with water.

- After allowing your skin to rest for about an hour, Aquafor or another petroleum jelly is applied to your skin; the petroleum jelly must stay in place for about 24 hours. A scabbing or crust will develop and you simply follow the instructions from your practitioner and all should be well[7].

Lash Treatments

Lastly, here's some information on how to get your eyelashes as full and voluptuous as Aunt Mabel's bosom. As we age, our eyelashes become thinner, shorter, and lighter - boo-hoo! On top of everything else, we have to worry about our eyelashes too? Well, yes.

Long, dark eyelashes make our eyes look bigger and younger. When we "dress up" lots of us apply temporary eyelash extensions or false eyelashes. Even more of us apply an extra coat of mascara to accentuate our eyes by outlining them with beautiful lashes. It's not fair that we lose our lashes, as we get older, just when we need them the most. It seems as though the lost eyelash hair comes back with a vengeance on our chins and upper lips – darn you Mother Nature! Never fear, there are some solutions to thinning, sparse lashes. Read on…

Revitalash, Neulash, LiLash and many other eyelash treatments are readily available over the counter with new eyelash products being released often. Some of these products are quite pricy where others are somewhat less expensive. The on-line reports from customers that use these products range from "It didn't do anything for me" to "Oh my god! My lashes are huge and thick in a couple of weeks!" Discussion of the over the counter lash products will not be included in this book because there are too many products and the results are too varied. The current *prescription* product available to consumers is called Latisse.

Latisse is approved by the FDA (Food and Drug Administration) for eyelash growth and is manufactured by Allergan, the same company that produces Botox and Juvederm. Latisse has clinical studies to support its' effects and the large majority of people who use Latisse regularly, have noticed a big difference in the length, darkening, and amount of their lashes[8]. People who have lost their lashes and even eyebrows to chemotherapy also use Latisse with fantastic results.

There are a couple of side effects that are fairly common although temporary; eye irritation and redness, slight darkening of the upper eyelid skin at the lash line (but who cares, most of us use eyeliner to accentuate that area of the eyelid anyway, right?). One side effect that has made a lot of people hesitant to try Latisse is the possibility of darkening of the iris (the colored part of the eye). Latisse contains a medication that is also used for glaucoma treatment and is dropped directly into the eye. A very small percentage of patients using this medication for glaucoma reported their iris darkened from the medication. Because Latisse contains the same medication but is not dropped directly into the eye every night, there is a minimal chance the iris could darken. Since the release of Latisse to the general public for eyelash growth, as of this writing, there have been zero reports of this side effect in anyone with light colored eyes[9]. That's right, zero. Lots of people who use Latisse (including the author) have light blue or green eyes and have been using it for years. It's pretty neat when people start complimenting you on your eyelashes. Yes, your eyelashes – who would have thought? Long lashes just make your eyes POP! For a complete list of side effects, you'll have to talk to your aesthetic practitioner or visit the Latisse website at www.latisse.com.

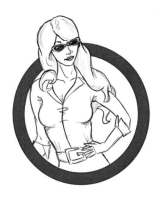

Chapter 4

THE MAGICAL THINGS WE CAN DO
WITH LIGHT, HEAT, AND BEING COOL

IPL: Reversing the damage you have done

Oh no! When you looked in the mirror this morning you realized your skin is not looking as perky and youthful as it once did back in the day, as we "over 40-ites" like to say. Too much fun in the sun when you were a teenager is costing you plenty. Why oh why is beauty wasted on the young? When we were teenagers, we looked in the mirror, and were certain that we were going to look this good and live-forever! As a matter of fact, we didn't even think about aging because we were too busy wondering how we could get our hair to look like Farrah Fawcett's without blowing a fuse in our mom and dad's house. Hey what just happened? It feels like we wake up one day and suddenly we're over 40! Or 50! What happened to our little bodies and our perfect skin?

Yes, we had perfect skin, unless acne was a frequent visitor and attacked you at the worst possible time in life – high school. High school was bad enough for most of us but to be blessed with those wonderful 2nd, 3rd, and 4th eyes just before "the dance" well, that was the cherry on the cake.

Speaking of cake, are those chocolate sprinkles on your face and chest or did you fall down in the parking lot? Oh, excuse me, its freckles from your gleeful times out at the beach enjoying your fantastic 20 something body and romping around in the sun all those years – goodness.

Before we get too caught up in the discussion of the fabulous IPL treatment detailed below, let's find out how wrinkly and photo-damaged we really are. Yes, there is a wrinkle scale that has been scientifically developed by Dr. Glogau and this is a slightly condensed version[1].

Type 1: No Wrinkles

Typical ages 20s – 30s
Early photoaging
Mild pigmentary changes
No or minimal wrinkles

Type 2: Wrinkles in Motion

Typical ages late 30s – 40s
Early to moderate photoaging
Moderate pigmentary changes, larger brown spots
Parallel smile lines beginning to appear to sides of mouth

Type 3: Wrinkles at Rest

Typical age 50s or older
Advanced photoaging
Obvious and numerous pigment changes/brown spots

Type 4: Only Wrinkles

Typical age 60 or older
Severe photoaging
Yellow-gray skin
Prior skin cancers
No normal skin

Keep in mind, you can look younger than your stated age on this scale if you have been good about protecting yourself from too much sun exposure and also have pretty good genes. For instance, you might be 45 but you are a Type 1 according to this scale. Nice isn't it? Alas, you can also look older than your stated age if you have been too sun exposed. For example, you can be 35 years old but be a Type 3 if you frequented tanning beds or baked yourself repeatedly out in the sun. Now let's get out there and turn ourselves into 1's! (OK, we can settle for 2's)...

Luckily for all of us, there is another magical treatment invented just for us previous sun worshipers. It's called Intense Pulsed Light or IPL. The name says it all – it is intense, it is pulsed, and it is a light, a very bright light. Nothing can prepare you for the actual treatment itself. The light is so bright that even with eye protection in the form of goggles or pads, the light can still be 'seen'. It's like when you blink as someone is taking your picture, you still see the flash – and flash it is! Secondly, when the pulse is delivered to your skin, you see the flash and you simultaneously feel a warm poke or snap. I admit, it's not as if you are getting a relaxing facial but the results are truly remarkable, seriously remarkable, majorly remarkable.

But seriously, Intense Pulsed Light (IPL) treatments are the gold standard for actually *reversing* sun damage and creating a more even skin tone and therefore, a more youthful appearance. IPL treatments stimulate collagen production; decreases the appearance of fine lines, sunspots, redness and vessels. The treatment consists of multiple pulses of intense light applied to the face, chest, neck, almost anywhere, even hands and the treatment takes about 10-15 minutes. There is no down time and patients can go back to work immediately depending on the intensity of the treatment.

You might be asking yourself, 'how does this work?' Well, this is where we need to get a little technical (you can skip this part if you like). First, the light is a broad band light, meaning it encompasses many wavelengths and colors of the light spectrum. You know the rainbow or prisms? Those colors are all *visible* light. Invisible light for example is x-rays, cosmic rays, microwaves, and infra-red[2]. Visible light is absorbed by chromophores in the skin, which is a fancy term for things that carry color such as blood or pigmented cells. When these chromophores absorb this special light, they become damaged and rise to the top layer of skin and slough off[3]. Your skin doesn't want it there as much as you don't want it there. In the case of those bothersome tiny blood vessels around your nose or that redness on your cheeks, the light is absorbed by the red blood cells and that damages those red cells then your skin and body flush them away. Blood cells and vessels are more difficult to treat and tend to grow back – boy our bodies are amazing aren't they? Annoying is more like it! Unfortunately, vessels and redness are like a perpetual harvest of sweet summer corn.

Here's How It Works:

- The fabulous IPL treatment begins on cleansed skin, with a cool, clear gel applied to the area to be treated.

- Dark goggles or eye pads will be given to you to protect your eyes from irritation.

- The smooth glass surface of the IPL crystal is gently applied to your skin and pulses of light are applied.

- A slight warm stinging sensation, like a snap of a small rubber band might be felt. Simultaneously, there is some sort of cooling mechanism during the treatment. Usually, the hand piece itself has an apparatus that cools the skin. Sometimes, an assistant is holding a cold air device directed at your skin, whereas others use plain old cold packs after treatment.

If you've already had one of these treatments, I know what you're thinking! An anesthetic cream may be used but is seldom required unless you have an extremely low pain tolerance or you are a man (wink, wink). Several treatments may be needed to achieve desired affects and the number of treatments depends on the severity of the problem. Unfortunately, if you suffer from rosacea or redness in your skin, you will likely need to receive IPL treatments periodically because there really is no "cure" for this, only management…sorry. The greatest benefits from IPL treatments are; significant reduction in uneven pigmentation, significant temporary reduction in redness from damaged veins and capillaries, reduced appearance of age brown spots or birthmarks, and can eliminate certain types of unwanted hair. Oh yes, and it also does dishes ☺

Costs for IPL treatments range in price from $99 - $450 each. Is there a downside, you ask? Not really. Treatments DO NOT cause cancer because IPL wavelengths are different than the sun's radiation wavelengths, and as a matter of fact, IPL is sometimes used to treat pre-cancerous lesions[4]. Wow! Noticeable cosmetic improvement can be seen within 1-2 weeks with immediate response occurring within minutes after the first treatment.

Radiofrequency and Ultrasound Devices Turn Up the Heat!

In our quest for tighter and smoother looking skin, the advent of devices that heat up collagen and result in some skin tightening have been developed. Unfortunately, the results are less than fantastic on some people. On the other hand, they work very well on other people and that's where a thorough consultation with an experienced clinician comes in handy. Part of the clinician's job is to educate and evaluate your skin and tell you if you are a good candidate for this type of procedure. Keep in mind, not everyone is a good candidate. You can give yourself a head start and whip out your mirror again and take a look at your face. Take a real hard look. Do you have skin that "hangs off" your jawline? You know, jowls? Do you have skin hanging off your neck that reminds your friends and relatives about Thanksgiving? If so, this procedure will likely not benefit you as much as a subtle, dare I say, face-lift by an experienced and thoughtful plastic surgeon. I know, I know, you don't want to go under the knife but that may be your only option at this point.

If you do not have skin hanging off your face and you have pretty good, plump, skin tone, you are a better candidate, although no promises. Why would someone with nice, tight skin need this procedure you ask? Well, we're not sure but maybe to give a little more of a lift or to temporarily prevent skin from sagging. Isn't it funny that the ones who don't really need the treatment get the best results? It's just not fair. The main thing is to realize that nothing works perfectly and your skin will not likely return to the era of when you were 20 and didn't have a skin care concern in the world!

So you have a better understanding of what these devices do and how they work let's take a look behind the scenes. You can also explore online and have a look at what's out there. Just be aware that a lot of the stories out there may be less than positive - actually about *any* cosmetic treatments. Again, the best path is to see an experienced aesthetic clinician that you feel good about and can trust with your skin.

There are several different models of skin tightening devices but the one you have probably heard of the most is Thermage. However, as of this writing, several others exist and are similar in their results so we won't address all of them but other popular models are Excilis, Polaris, Titan, Reaction, SkinTyte, Ulthera, and Accent. Some of these types of devices also are used to tighten skin on the belly, arms, knees and other body areas that tend to make their way south.

The data shows in un-biased studies[5,6] shows that less than 50% of the patients were satisfied with their treatment results as far as improving sagging skin. However, other studies[7,8] have shown that younger patients, say under 50 years old, and patients who receive two or more treatments, and/or two or more passes with the hand-piece, are more satisfied than those who endure only one treatment. Keep in mind, these treatments can be costly, averaging about $2000 per treatment and may be higher or lower according to body part, number of passes, time involved, or other variables specific to the office policy of the place you choose to receive treatments.

The scientific evidence suggests the heat from the device heats up the collagen fibers in the skin and causes the skin to contract and build more collagen. The superficial layers of skin are not damaged in any way but only the deeper layers are heated and respond to treatment. Since the epidermis is not affected, there is zero decrease in pigment (brown spots) so this is not an effective treatment for decreasing sunspots or other pigments in the skin. This is the same whether a radio frequency (i.e. Thermage) or Infra red (i.e. Titan) device is used. Controlled deep heat = collagen stimulation but no pigment improvement.

Theoretically, the heat from the radio frequency or infrared treatment affects the skin and it thinks it has been injured (tortured is more like it from what some patients report). Then the skin does its natural process of trying to heal itself and voila! Tighter skin, hopefully.

Pain control varies and can include topical numbing cream and/or injections that numb the area, along with oral medications such as Valium or Vicodin. You will relax for a short amount of time, usually 30 – 45 minutes before the procedure, to let the medication(s) take effect. The average length of time treating the face is about 45 minutes. The procedure itself has been described as less than comfortable; some say it is downright painful. Noticeable tightening of the skin can take up to 6 months so it is not immediately gratifying as some of the other treatments previously described. Please get a thorough consultation prior to signing up...

Two Words of Advice

First - Now, don't take this the wrong way but don't wait too long to begin getting some kind of aesthetic treatments and/or procedures. If you do, you will likely be very disappointed at what might be available to you when you finally decide to start looking better and improving the quality of your skin and appearance. This is not a sales pitch, this is real information based on many years of experience with many different types of people wanting many different types of results. Make it easy on yourself and don't learn the hard way, if you're curious or distressed about your appearance, start looking at options right away.

Women come in everyday hoping to reverse the clock in one day or with one treatment to un-do years and years of damage and abuse to their skin. This is not a realistic approach. Sometimes your skin has just given up and is sadly hanging on you, all wrinkly and thin from sun damage, smoking, the natural aging process, and/or chronic neglect. You shouldn't expect to come in looking like a prune and leave looking like a plum!

Many people are hesitant to start using the treatment options available nowadays because of a variety of reasons such as cost, fear of the outcome, stigma of "having work done", cynicism, and others. This book provides you with information so you can feel comfortable exploring your options sooner rather than later. Little bits at a time, baby steps – that's all you need. For example, start with a microdermabrasion and an IPL to even out the appearance of your skin and reverse some of the sun damage and brown spots you might have. Then after you see those results, maybe dabble in a Botox or Dysport treatment to smooth out the lines on your forehead or around your eyes. Just with those suggestions, you will notice a wonderful and rejuvenated improvement in your appearance. People will ask you what you've been doing - "A new cream? Vacation? Diet? Haircut?" They won't be able to figure it out; you'll just look better – not different.

Second – Don't take this the wrong way either but you can be pretty young and start getting aesthetic treatments. Obviously, teenagers can get the photodynamic therapy for acne treatment, facials, and microdermabrasions for overall skin care. But what about Botox? Dysport? Fillers? Well, some 19 and 20 year olds have inherited things from their moms and dads or even grandma and grandpa for that matter. Deep lines on the forehead or in between the eyebrows from strong muscle movement start to appear. These lines tend to bother younger people the same way they bother older people and the younger people (18+ years old) are perfectly fine to receive Botox or Dysport to help smooth those lines before they turn into crevices that may need a small amount of filler to correct later. Or maybe they've inherited thin lips and would like a little more volume – that's fine too. This is not to say that people under 20 years old should run out and get aesthetic treatments, but it is nice to know they certainly can and do!

Just remember, the effects of aesthetic treatments don't last forever and you do need to take care of your skin but it is so nice we have these options available to us. And don't worry, once you start doing aesthetic treatments, you don't have to continue if you don't want to or if you have a change in financial status. You can discontinue anytime without repercussions to your skin. You can start anytime too.

The vast majority of people who step slowly and gently into the world of aesthetic treatments (and even those who jump in with both feet) tend to stay there. It's comfy and it makes you feel great because you look great. It's like your own little magical world. Enjoy exploring and welcome!

Warning! Everything doesn't always come up roses.

Hold everything! Before you throw down this book and run out to have one of these fabulous IPL or laser hair reduction treatments you need to do a little research on the office and the clinician who will actually be doing your treatment. There is nothing wrong with having one practitioner sit down and speak with you about the treatment and then have another one actually do the treatment, but you must be clear on the credentials of anyone who is going to touch your face. It's your face for goodness sake! Just because a practitioner has some fancy initials behind their name doesn't automatically make them an expert. Some significant side effects such as hyperpigmentation (worsening of your brown spots), burns, or scars have occurred when inexperienced or too aggressive clinicians are performing these treatments. Proper training, knowledge, and respect for the skin are essential for fabulous results no matter who is performing your treatments.

Here are some questions to ask:

❖ Are you a registered nurse (RN), aesthetician, medical doctor (MD, DO), doctor of nursing practice (DNP), nurse practitioner (NP) or physician assistant (PA)? If they answer yes, depending on the state you live in, you're making progress. If they answer, "I'm the receptionist", "I'm the consultant" or "I'm the accountant" don't walk away – RUN!

❖ How long have you been doing these treatments?

❖ Where did you receive your training?

❖ How many of these treatments have you done? (This is a good question because you can determine if they have experience and how much).

One thing to keep in mind, being the good patient you are, you do not want to alienate your practitioner right off the bat, or at all for that matter. Hurling these questions at her during your first meeting can put her on edge and not set the mood for an enjoyable experience. Best to let her know you are a rational person and hope she understands you care about your skin, that's why you're in her office. You could also let her know you've done your research and have chosen her office because you feel comfortable there. Additionally, it might be wise to visit their website and scan for credentials and experience. In any case, please be choosy about who touches your face, neck, or chest.

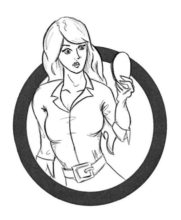

Chapter 5

BOTOX, DYSPORT, AND OTHER BOTULINUM TOXINS TYPE A'S

Freeze! You're Gorgeous!

Ok, this is a favorite treatment of millions of beautiful men and women. My god, we can't live without this stuff. Ah, Botox, magical Botox; you're so wonderful someone should write a song about you…and your cousins Dysport (pronounced dis-port), Myobloc, and Xeomin. These are truly amazing treatments for lines and wrinkles. They are so fabulous that some creams are marketing themselves as "better than Botox". Really?! Because we'd all love to be able to rub on a cream and have it do the same wonderful things to our skin that Botox, Dysport and other type-A toxins can do. This sounds just like the promises of cellulite creams and massages – wouldn't it be awesome to have your cheesy cellulite rubbed, or better yet, wiped off? Oh sweet baby Jo-Jo, sign us up!!

The Botox and Dysport medications are made from a purified form of the botulinum toxin. They work by blocking the neuromuscular transmission through binding to acceptor sites on motor nerve terminals, and inhibiting the release of acetylcholine[1]. Ok, say that three times fast. Basically, it prevents the chemical reaction necessary to move the muscle. It only works on the *motor* nerves, not the sensory nerves so yes, if someone slaps you on the forehead, you will feel it.

When these medications are injected into the target muscle, at correct doses, they produce nice smooth skin by reducing the muscle activity. Muscle contraction is what causes the lines between your eyebrows, across your forehead, and around your eyes. Botox et al. is not good for treating lines that are caused from sun damage or volume loss (see fillers and IPL).

These medications are currently administered using a tiny needle that goes into the skin. This treatment is virtually painless and requires no anesthetic. Do not concern yourself with thoughts of a needle poking you in the face – really. These needles are so tiny they use bigger ones on babies! Also, they do not go so deep that they hit your brain; the skull is there to protect your brain, besides, the needle is so small and fine it would bend and break if someone tried to push it anywhere near your brain. Some people get so nervous about a "needle going in my face" that they don't think logically. It's kind of cute, a tiny bit unreasonable, but cute.

Ok, the entire treatment takes about 3 minutes and you're done. There hasn't been one person I've treated that hasn't said, "That's it?" Seriously. However, the effects of the Botox or Dysport take anywhere from 2 – 10 days to reach full potential so you don't have to worry about waking up one morning with a suddenly flawless face, it takes a few days. Everyone responds pretty similarly to these medications but some people need a little tweak after their first time – some, not at all. It's always a good idea to see your practitioner about 2 weeks after your first treatment so they can see your results and answer any new questions you may have. On rare occasions, you may need a touch up at that follow-up appointment to give you perfect results for your unique face. If that's the case, you will likely start out at the same dose next time. Oh yes, there will be a next time because you will love the result if it's done correctly.

Speaking of taking a few days, there are over the counter topical creams out there touting the same miraculous effects as Botox and Dysport. Gee, if these over the counter creams really worked, we'd all put down those friendly syringes and tiny needles and reach for these fabulous little jars, wouldn't we?

Actually, there is a pharmaceutical company, Revance Therapeutics (www.revance.com), in the late phases of clinical trials looking into a topical prescription gel that may mimic the effects of Botox and Dysport. It appears the effects are working pretty well on the thin skin around the eyes but not so much on other areas of the face. The idea behind this gel is to help the small percentage of people who are needle-phobic but would still like the smoothing effects of Botox or Dysport get the treatment. This novel gel is applied to the skin and left in place for about 30 minutes, then washed off; the effects last about three to four months. They are getting good results on the underarm area as well for treatment of excessive sweating but it looks like its years away from market. Here's a tissue. ☹

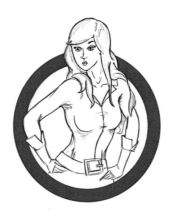

Chapter 6

FILLERS: GET THOSE LIPS AND CHEEKS BACK WHERE THEY BELONG!

Dermal Fillers

There are many FDA approved dermal fillers on the U.S. market today. They include collagen, Perlane, Restylane, Juvederm, Sculptra, Artefill, Radiesse, silicone, and autologous (your own) fat. Typically, there are one or more fillers in clinical trials at any given time as well as new ones released onto the marketplace periodically. The focus of this chapter will not include the permanent fillers of silicone and autologous fat; those are reserved for our magical colleagues, the plastic surgeons. Yes, it's true! You can take fat from your butt and put it in your face.

Here you will learn about the common temporary fillers that all of your friends are getting, the ones that last less than 5 years (fillers, not your friends lasting less than 5 years). Since the temporary dermal fillers are made of different substances, they will be discussed according to substance and also trade name.

Collagen

The first filler we will look at briefly is collagen. Collagen used to be the 'gold standard' after it got approved in the 80's although it has been studied since the 50's. What we learned is that collagen didn't last very long, only about 3 months. This fueled a quest for longer lasting, affordable, formulations that did not migrate[1]. This new and exciting formulation was hyaluronic acid or the hylans. Hip-hip-hooray!

The Hylans

There are many hylans on the global market but the most common ones used in the U.S. at the moment are Perlane, Restylane, and Juvederm and their special sub-classes i.e. Restylane-L (with lidocaine), Juvederm XC (with lidocaine), Juvederm Ultra, etc. They are all hylans; that is, they are derivatives of hyaluronic acid, which is a naturally occurring substance in our skin and bodies. Products available here and elsewhere are packaged in pre-filled syringes. The clinician has no control on the amount contained in each syringe, however patient and clinician, have full control of *how many* syringes to use. The syringes contain 0.5 mL to 2 mL, with the 1 mL syringe containing an amount about the size of a petite ladies' little finger. Some patients' need only one to correct their issue, others need more.

These fillers are wonderful for plumping up our thinning lips, cheeks, temples, and the droopy corners of our mouth, sunken hollows under our eyes, jawline, and even our hands. Hylans usually last 6 - 12 months[2] in the face and about 6 – 8 months[3] in the lips initially. They are water-soluble, and slowly reabsorbed into the skin. These fillers appear to last longer and longer upon repeated use with some people reporting they last 2 years or more!

The treatments nowadays are so much more comfortable than they used to be. In the old days, there was a significant amount of discomfort, well let's be honest, pain and some people said, "I'll never do that again!" The conundrum was, many loved the result so much that they prolonged repeating their treatment due to fear but eventually endured the torture yet again. Then, many kind and loving clinicians began using a dental block to numb the lips. Yes, the same thing your dentist does to you but you don't look as good after she/he's done. Patients endured the dental block discomfort to get their fabulous lips but it sure made the treatment more comfortable. So what if you were slobbering and drooling on the way out – you looked fantastic!

Thankfully, most manufacturers now create their hylan formulations to include a numbing component contained inside it without sacrificing the amount of product. All we do now is apply a topical numbing cream, let you sit for a few short minutes, do the painless treatment and "voila!" – luscious lips or cheeks or both!

All you feel is the initial poke of the tiny needle, that's 'about it'. 'About it' because some injectors are gentler than others, it's all in the technique dahling. Marvelous...

Of course, anytime a needle goes through your skin, whether you're getting a flu shot, donating blood, or getting your lips done, you have a chance of getting a bruise. Occasionally people get a small bruise, whereas less often they can get a real honker. Usually, a bruise is no big deal but when it happens on your face, it seems to carry more mystery, embarrassment, and intrigue. People look at a man with a small bruise on his face and wonder if he hit his face on the car door (or someone's fist?). People look at a woman with a small bruise on her face and wonder if she had 'work done' – it's just not fair, sniff, sniff.

There are no guarantees you will bruise, and there are no guarantees you won't, but you can do a few things to help prevent bruising. First, do not drink alcohol 24 hours prior to your treatment. Yes, alcohol thins your blood and makes for easy bruising. Second, do not take aspirin or other blood thinners like ibuprofen 4 – 7 days prior to your treatment unless you take them for heart conditions then please continue. Third, if you bruise easily, you can take a homeopathic remedy called Arnica Montana. It really works.

Some bruises are barely noticeable whereas others can last a week or two. This has nothing to do with the skill of your clinician but has everything to do with that little needle puncturing the tiny blood vessel unseen beneath the skin. Believe me, if we could see every vessel, no one would ever get a bruise. Then there's the swelling, oh, and probably some temporary redness. Swelling occurs in most people but people with seasonal allergies tend to swell a bit more than people without allergies. If swelling does happen, it usually lasts for a maximum of 48 hours and is usually not super noticeable. Similarly, redness is not very significant and usually resolves within hours.

Rarely is anyone allergic to these types of fillers although one study found some patients who had an allergic response but it was less than 0.4% of the population[4]. Now, there are some bad things that can happen with fillers. Sometimes if the product is placed too close to the surface of the skin, you can see it. Alternatively, if it is placed too deeply, it doesn't last as long as it should. Additionally, there are more serious side effects (although rare) of vascular compromise that can lead to scarring. All of these things and more can be addressed with your clinician during the consultation.

Now for the good stuff about fillers. You can enhance your looks so easily and be as subtle or dramatic as you and your practitioner decide. Most women absolutely love their lips and/or cheeks (etc.) after treatment with appropriate filler; they wish they had done it sooner. These treatments give an incredible lift, not just to their spirits but also to their faces! Not only do these women look better and more refreshed, they *feel* it. This is one reason over 12 million cosmetic treatments were performed in 2011 and the number grows steadily[5].

Of course we have all seen someone who has gone a little too far or maybe a lot too far. These people scare us, all of us. Scary comes in many different forms; lips that look like they're trying to escape the face, cheeks that are so swollen they appear to be full of marshmallows, and eyes that, well, we can't quite pinpoint the problem. Don't worry about looking strange because you have learned that you have as much say in your appearance as the practitioner and together you will decide how you would like to look.

If you have full lips and want just a little more plumpness then voila! That is what you will get. Just remember, they will still be your lips, just a little plumper. If you have very thin, skinny lips there is definitely help for you too it just takes a bit more finesse, patience, and time. To get a natural look, we have to slowly build your lips up over time so you don't look like a duck or gorilla. Now, you can't have Angelina Jolie lips if you were born with teeny, tiny lips. Most likely giant lips wouldn't fit with the finer features on your face anyway.

Fillers will increase the size and change the shape of your lips but will add minimal 'color'. In other words, the lips can be adjusted a little bit so they turn up and show a little more of the colored part, but there are limits. If you have a wide smile, you can make your lips pouty. If you have a narrow smile, you can widen it a bit too. If you have a scar or other asymmetry, fillers can improve them as well. Fillers are truly magical!

The usual amount placed in lips during a treatment is 1 mL but there are exceptions. If you are too nervous and decide you only want a little bit and use less than a full 1 mL syringe, it usually makes a difference but not much of one. Then after a few days, you get used to your new look and it's barely noticeable. Most women return for an additional touch up if they use only 0.5mL. Do yourself a favor and jump in with both lips (you know what I mean).

The cheeks are a different story. The cheeks usually take 2 - 5 mL, using one or more 1 mL syringes on each side to start and this amount can make a nice difference by giving us the 'lift' many of us are looking for. However, depending on your skin, volume loss, and face shape, you might take more or less product than your friends and neighbors. Yes it's expensive and sounds like a lot of product but its really not (it takes 5 mL to make a teaspoon). Another bonus is that the hyaluronic acid fillers in the face can last about a year or even longer, especially with repeated treatments so at least you're not getting these treatments very often, maybe yearly. Come to think of it, you can schedule your annual filler appointment at the same time you schedule your mammogram or pelvic exam - how fun!

Cheek enhancement is a nice way to get a lift without undergoing the surgical knife. Even if you have waited too long and now need a facelift, you'll still look better if you add some youthful plumpness to your cheeks. The treatment is surprisingly easy.

Here's How It Works:

- After you have filled out the necessary paperwork, have had your consultation, and are nice and comfy in the treatment room, the clinician will review the process with you and likely take a "before photo".

- Then your skin will be cleansed either with alcohol or some other antibacterial cleanser and then a topical anesthetic will be applied to the area to be treated. The topical anesthetic is a prescription cream that is applied so there's no extra poking with more needles.

- After the topical anesthetic has had a chance to work, usually 10 – 30 minutes depending on the medications used, it is wiped off and your skin is cleaned with alcohol.

- Now for the fun part, no really, it's not bad at all. As a matter of fact, there is usually zero pain associated with fillers in this treatment area. The product is gently injected into the skin with a very thin needle or cannula and in about 15 – 30 minutes depending on the clinician, your treatment is done.

(➜Note: Speed of the procedure has nothing to do with the outcome; some people are slower, more methodical injectors whereas others are very fast and accurate. More often than not, the more experienced injectors are a bit faster but usually not by much so it's hard to tell just from the time it takes to get your lift if your injector is experienced or not: see Chapter 4, under questions to ask).

- After you are done, the clinician or assistant will give you ice packs or some other cooling agent and you should sit for a few minutes while your skin cools. Cooling helps with swelling and bruising, however most people get a little pink or red where the ice has been held after a few minutes.

- Then, the "after photo" is likely taken and you will be on your merry way in no time. Straight to the check out counter where you will part with some of your cash that has been burning a hole in your pocket (book).

Pricing will vary depending on a variety of things; the amount of product you use, the state/county/city/region where you have been treated, experience of injector, location of office i.e. within a TV star plastic surgeon's office vs. a beauty salon (yikes!), etc. A price list of common ranges is found in Chapter 12.

Sculptra

Sculptra is not generally regarded as "dermal filler" because it is made from polymerized lactic acid (PLA) that is similar to what sutures are made from. This material is mixed with sterile water and typically an anesthetic such as lidocaine[6]. Unfortunately for most of us, we would like instant results and sadly, Sculptra takes weeks to months before noticeable improvement is seen. On average, 3 treatments are required and the results should be noticeable after approximately 6 weeks. However, in some people this may take longer or require more treatments.

There is some initial swelling that occurs right after the treatment however it eventually goes away, leaving you to think the product may not have worked. Never fear, Sculptra is different. This product actually stimulates dermal connective tissue regeneration through, well no one is exactly sure how, but the skin responds beautifully and you get the fullness you've wanted; you might have to wait a little longer. The results typically last a couple of years or even longer. This product is not used in lips or some other areas of the face, depending on what your issue might be though; you can discuss it with your practitioner. Plastic surgeons, among others, love this stuff.

Radiesse

Radiesse is another temporary filler that works by replacing lost volume through a gel that contains tiny microspheres of calcium hydroxylapatite (bone mineral). After the product is injected into the skin, the gel is absorbed and the spheres cause a reaction so the skin produces collagen. The microspheres are composed of the same material that bone and tissue are formed. The effects of the modern formulation last about a year or even longer. Some studies have demonstrated the need for repeat treatments prior to a year to maintain effect and longevity[7,8]. This product should be placed deeply into the skin if used in naso-labial folds or it can be seen. Sometimes this product is placed into the cheeks or hands but should not be used in lips, under eyes, or certain other areas. Many practitioners love Radiesse and use it often so product choice is up to you and the practitioner; talk amongst yourselves.

Artefill/Artecoll

This is permanent dermal filler, and is made from polymethylmethacrylate (PMMA) beads in a collagen vehicle. PMMA is a transparent thermoplastic that has many uses, among them as permanent filler. What happens in the skin after injection with this substance is the collagen is absorbed after a couple of months and the PMMA beads cause a foreign body reaction (basically your body forms fibrous tissue around the beads) resulting in very long lasting fullness[9]. One thing to consider with permanent filers is that as you age and your face changes over time, the fillers may not look as natural as they did at the time they were placed. This is yet another decision you can discuss with your practitioner, remember, you are involved with your face too.

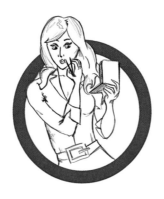

Chapter 7

LASERS, HAIR REMOVAL, AND SKIN RESURFACING: GO TO THE LIGHT

Light is magic too.

Laser light is an incredible phenomenon. This magical light is transformed into heat in the body, skin, or hair shaft. Depending on the depth of penetration for the desired treatment, the laser beam basically travels through crystal, liquid or gas. For example, the CO_2 laser beams travel through CO_2 gas whereas the Ruby laser beam goes through a ruby colored crystal[1]. Depending on the depth and target structure that absorbs the laser beam, it determines which structures absorb the heat and are damaged, (i.e. hair follicle, brown pigment, veins, water). Pretty neat, huh?

Laser Hair Removal (Reduction)
Goodbye Razor!

Do you remember when you asked, well let's be honest, more like *begged* your mom to let you shave your legs? Underarms? Arms? Do you remember her saying "Once you start, you'll never stop"? But you didn't care. Your best friend at school gets to shave. You should be able to shave too. After all, you're almost an adult!

Now I'll bet you're kicking yourself thinking that all of your shaving made this dark, coarse, manly hair grow at the speed of light. Not so. Not even close. You see hair grows from the inside of your skin outward. The hair follicle living in your skin produces hair cells that build on top of one another until they poke out through a pore. Shaving hair, any hair, will not make it grow in any thicker or change the color. If that were true, balding men would shave their heads and sport full heads of hair!

Many people are bothered by excess hair growing in places they wish it wasn't. For example, the chin, the upper lip, the legs, the underarms, and the bikini line – you get the picture. The lasers used for laser hair removal work by converting laser energy into heat. This heat travels down the hair shaft and is absorbed by the melanin (colored cells) in your hair. The more melanin in the hair shaft, the more heat is absorbed by the hair and the more heat reaches the follicle. This heat distorts or destroys the hair follicle so it can't produce another hair. Or the hair it does produce is pretty wimpy – light and fine[2]. This is the reason it is now called permanent "Laser Hair Reduction"

90

(LHR) instead of permanent laser hair removal. It was decided by our friends (attorneys), labeling this treatment as permanent hair removal, is misleading since some hairs may grow back, albeit wimpy (as above).

That being said, if you do not have enough melanin in your hair, the laser will not work. For example, lasers do not work on blonde, grey, or light brown hair. Why? There is not enough pigmented cells, or melanin, in the hair to absorb the heat. You can pout and scream and cry but those grey hairs poking out of your chin will not respond to laser. They *will* respond to electrolysis, however.

Electrolysis is a treatment performed by aestheticians, cosmetologists, electrologists, and others that uses a fine needle to introduce an electric current directly into the hair follicle to destroy the hair where it grows, like laser, only different. Electrolysis results do not depend on the color of the hair, any hair color responds to electrolysis because the needle is introduced directly into the follicle[3]. This procedure requires more of a time commitment and many sessions to complete a small area but it is wonderful for permanent hair reduction in people who do not have hair types that respond to laser. For many hair reduction candidates, laser hair reduction treatments are superior to electrolysis due to the speed and effectiveness of today's lasers.

Back to the laser we go for some hair reduction. There are several types of lasers used for hair reduction, all of which are effective if the combination of hair color, density, skin type, and clinician expertise are appropriate.

Some lasers are better for darker skin than others (i.e. Nd:YAG 1064nm laser or long pulsed alexandrite 755nm) although different, gentler settings on most lasers will do just fine. There are more risks of burns and pigment changes on darker skinned individuals so keep this in mind if you have darker skin. This doesn't mean you cannot get laser treatments for hair reduction, it just means you need to be aware of the potential problems and should discuss any light or laser based treatments with your practitioner.

The same is true for people with tanned skin; there is more risk for burns and pigment changes. Yes, you can receive laser treatments but you will have to endure more treatments because the energy needs to be decreased or turned down to avoid burns. It's better, more efficient, more effective, and safer to be as pale as you can be before you start and during your treatments. Also, if you don't time it perfectly and get your first one or two treatments right before you start tanning for summer, don't worry. You can resume your treatments again after summer if you need to wait. The hair follicles that were destroyed will not produce another hair so the process won't reverse if you need to take a break for a few months. However you will notice other hairs will grow back if they were not hit in the growth phase during the initial treatments. Sometimes these hairs go into 'shock', take longer to regenerate, and show up later. This does not mean your treatments were ineffective, it just means you'll need to resume treatments as soon as you are nice and pale and paste-y. Neat-o!

The treatment is not real comfortable, some would say it's nothing at all and others would say it is downright excruciating depending on the area of the body being treated. Some people say, the bikini line, is worse than the underarms. Some say the reverse. And some say the upper lip is more painful than the areolas (the colored part around the nipples). Others say the reverse. Some people feel like they're getting a massage, others feel like they are having a baby – pain perception really swings wide. Everyone has a different pain tolerance; different people tolerate the procedure more easily than others. The sensation of laser hair removal has been described as feeling like "being poked with hot needles", "being sprinkled with hot water", "being pecked to death by a chicken", "torture", "oh, it's not that bad" "ticklish" along with other colorful remarks. The thing is, the results are so good that it is worth it for many people. And remember, waxing is not that pleasant and you have to do that forever. Think of the money you'll save on razors and waxing appointments if you get laser treatments instead.

Actually there are some less painful lasers in use today. There is a high-speed laser that is much faster and much more comfortable than previous lasers used for hair reduction called the Lumenis High Speed Lightsheer (see www.skinandhealth.com for more information on this device). This laser works through the same principles as other lasers but it has a much larger treatment spot size and utilizes vacuum assist technology that makes the treatment much more comfortable than traditional hair removal lasers. The bonus about this particular laser is that your underarms, yes both underarms, are done in about 3 minutes, both lower legs including the knees are done in about 20 minutes – it's true! Treatment with this laser has been described as "a pinch and a warm poke", "hot pressure", "a pull and a snap".

The treatment with any type of laser for hair removal follows the same laser physics because of the characteristics of the hair itself. You will need multiple treatments in the same area, i.e. underarms, spaced several weeks to months apart depending on the area because the hair grows in three phases. Unfortunately, the laser only works in one of those three phases, anagen or, the growth phase, that's why you have to endure multiple treatments; usually a minimum of 5 treatments spaced 4 – 6 weeks apart. After the sessions are completed, it is highly likely you will need to visit your practitioner periodically for maintenance treatments anywhere from 6 months to every couple of years. Hey, it beats shaving every day! The three phases of hair growth are:

1) anagen – where the hair is actively growing out of the follicle

2) catagen – where the hair is done growing and is now "resting" and

3) telogen – where the hair is shedding or coming out of the body.

What is so interesting is, hair in different body areas, have genetic programs that determine how long each growth stage is and to what length the hair will grow. For example, hair on the scalp can be in the anagen or growing phase for 2 – 8 years whereas the hair of the eyebrows is in the growing phase for only 2 – 3 months. Another aspect to consider is hairs in the telogen or shedding phase also vary depending on the body region. For example the shedding phase is occurring in only 5 – 15% of scalp hairs at one time vs. 40 – 50% of hairs on the trunk[4]. So, the hairs on the trunk, for instance bikini line or underarms, are in the shedding phase almost half the time. Remember, the laser does not work in this phase, only the growth phase. Ah-ha! That's why you need multiple treatments!

Although it is not a one-time treatment, most people love the results of having baby smooth skin and no razor burn, especially before summer. If you suffer from ingrown hairs, especially after shaving, laser hair reduction is a very effective treatment for them. Yes, it works wonderfully on ingrown hairs, and will make them so much better. You won't believe it! And whatever you do, do not pick at those ingrown hairs whether or not you are getting laser treatments. As you probably already know, you'll be left with unsightly scars and pick marks and no one wants that!

The most popular areas that are treated with lasers for hair removal are; the underarms, bikini line, legs, back, and that little hair trail from the pubic area to the belly button. Other areas commonly treated include the upper lip and chin in women, beard and moustache areas in men, areolas, chest, toes, ears…wait a minute, almost any area can be treated. Let's list exceptions instead; vagina (va-jay-jay), anus, inside the nose, eyelashes and any area where there is a mucous membrane involved. Now you might be thinking, 'Hold on, my friend had her entire bikini line done where ALL of her hair is gone; she's bald as an eagle! What do you mean I can't have mine done too?' Well, yes you may have your entire bikini line done, but you cannot have the vagina done. There's no hair in there anyway, same with the anus. Oh there might be gobs of hair *around* those areas but not in them. If those areas burn and scar, there may be dysfunction and no one wants a dysfunctional anus! Although, we might work for one.

Other Methods of Hair Removal

In case you are not relishing the laser for hair removal, there are a few other options; electrolysis as previously mentioned, waxing, shaving, tweezing, and Intense Pulsed Light (IPL). The IPL is used for hair reduction as well as photo-rejuvenation. Since we are all experts at waxing, shaving and tweezing those methods will not be reviewed here. However, IPL is a popular method for hair reduction and it works in the same way as lasers.

The IPL has different wavelengths that are absorbed by different structures, hair cells and hair follicles being two of them. As with the lasers, the IPL must be absorbed by chromophores (colored targets) within the desired area of treatment. The best results occur when the hair is dark and the skin is light. The IPL heat is absorbed by the hair, travels to the hair follicle, and damages the follicle. Isn't that wonderful? Ah-ha, you may think this way doesn't hurt as much as the laser, but alas, you're incorrect, wrong...unfortunately IPL doesn't tickle.

Laser Skin Resurfacing – Like Buttah

Here we'll look at the popular fractional lasers used in treatment for skin rejuvenation. In the early 2000s, the development of fractional lasers changed the approach to laser skin rejuvenation. Fractional lasers produce numerous, microscopic, beams of laser light that treat only a defined fraction of the skin within a targeted area, leaving tiny areas of skin unaffected. Get it? Fraction = fractional... Imagine a ½ inch square filled with a hundred tiny dots. This is one pattern used to do these types of treatments. Those tiny dots are where the laser touched and in between those dots is your untouched skin. Your untouched skin allows for rapid recovery by sending new, healing cells to the wounded areas[5].

The non-ablative fractional lasers include the 2940 nm fractional erbium:yttrium (pronounced "huh?") aluminum garnet (Er:YAG) laser, the 2790 nm fractional yttrium scandium gallium (pronounced "what-tha?") garnet (YSGG) laser. The 10,600 nm fractional CO_2 laser is ablative which means it goes a little deeper into the dermis. Wow, you can say that again! Some popular models you may have heard of are DOT Smartxide, Fraxel, Deep FX, and Starlux among others.

But don't be scared, these days the lasers used for skin rejuvenation are not the completely ablative ones you've heard about that left a line of demarcation around the jawline - young face above and turkey neck below.

97

That's because the delicate skin of the neck couldn't tolerate those intense, fully ablative treatments very well. The fractional laser treatments most commonly used today have a much easier and shorter healing time and great results.

The laser beam used for resurfacing skin works like magic. The laser actually ablates (vaporizes) the skin where it touches leaving a very tiny dotted pattern over the surface that's being treated; face, neck, chest, hands, etc. Heat is delivered to the skin and causes shrinkage and tightening of the skin while at the same time stimulating the fibroblasts (collagen producing cells) in the skin that make more collagen[6].

The effect of the fractional laser resurfacing is one of total rejuvenation with removal of surface brown and red marks and reduction in acne scars, skin laxity, lines and wrinkles while giving you an overall appearance of smoother, more youthful skin[7]. Now, we don't get this wonderful effect without any down time, no, no. There are a few days of less than fun times. You're not oozing and bleeding and confined to your bed, but you will not want to go the mall either. There's usually some swelling, redness, and sometimes pinpoint bleeding. Most people experience some itching around day 3 that can be kind of annoying – oh and then there's the layer of petroleum jelly you have to wear on your skin for a couple of days. And also, there's peeling for a few days after the treatment as well. Very glamorous!

You may be wondering, does this procedure hurt? Well, in a word, yes. But, to control pain, the usual protocol is to have a topical anesthetic applied about one hour before the treatment. In addition, many offices will add some type of pain pill like Ibuprofen or Vicodin, and maybe one for anxiety as well, like Xanax, at the time the topical anesthetic is applied. HINT: If you have ever had a "cold sore" or herpes simplex virus (HSV), you should absolutely receive a prophylactic antiviral medication and take it the day prior to treatment, the day of treatment, and then for a few days afterwards to prevent a nasty breakout. Not everyone with the virus will get a recurrence but it's better to be safe than sorry.

On a more serious note, there can be some side effects, although they are not common and most are rare. These include infection, hyper- or hypo-pigmentation, scarring, or prolonged redness. All of these issues would be discussed with you in detail during your consultation. Other potential complications of fractional ablative laser resurfacing include temporary acne breakout, and milia (those tiny little white spots like on babies skin), but these can be easily treated[8].

Darker complexions have sun damage less often than lighter skinned folks and it is usually less severe to boot. Laser induced hyper- or hypo-pigmentation is a major concern in the darker skinned population, as the risk for this adverse effect increases in those with more skin pigmentation. Clinicians resurfacing for skin rejuvenation in patients with darker skin types prefer to use fractional ablative or traditional Er:YAG lasers in this subgroup of patients[9].

OK, not everyone is a candidate for the fractional laser treatments, but many people are great candidates. *Unsuitable* candidates may be tanned, have skin cancer in the area to be treated, had radiation therapy, form keloid scars, among other things. You would be smart to have a thorough consultation with the practitioner. The consultation would include things such as expected treatment outcome and skin improvement, anticipated recovery time, and risks.

Patients treated with the fractional CO_2 laser can usually return to normal activity after 5 to 10 days, depending on the intensity of treatment; less time is needed for recovery after fractional Er:YAG resurfacing. Depending on the concerns of the patient, skin quality, and desired effects, one to three treatments, is required.

Although laser resurfacing can lead to improvements in lines and wrinkles in the lip area, cheeks, and eye areas, deep nasolabial creases, marionette lines, and severe skin laxity are often best managed with treatments such as injectable dermal fillers (Ch. 6) and surgery (Ch. 9). Additionally, those pesky dynamic lines caused from muscle movement may come back after a successful fractional laser treatment and those are best kept under control with your new best friend and mine, Botox! Yes, we all wish there was one magic potion to take care of all of our woes. Some of us are luckier than others...

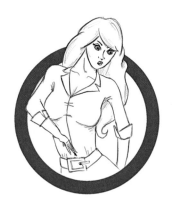

Chapter 8

PESKY CELLULITE AND FAT TREATMENTS

Why Won't it Just Go Away?

Wouldn't it be a glorious thing if we could lie on a comfortable table and have someone rub our fat or cellulite off our bodies? Or maybe have a series of injections to dissolve our fat and melt it away? It would be a dream come true! Some people declare they get great results from these types of treatments and their fat/cellulite is gone – how miraculous!

There are some products and treatments available now that claim this very thing and actually do work for a small, select group of people. These treatments are called endermologie, mesotherapy or lipo-dissolve. There are also topical potions but there are too numerous to mention here but can easily be searched on-line. The science behind these applications appear to be thin at best but theoretically these treatments and products should work; patient satisfaction can be less than optimal and most results are temporary. Additionally, the *unbiased* research doesn't support the majority of these treatments[1,2,3]. But, since there is an interest in non-surgical fat/cellulite reduction, it will be briefly described here.

Endermologie

Endermologie is a treatment that utilizes pressure and massage to "break up" the stringy bands that a few experts believe cause cellulite. These so-called bands theoretically pull the skin inward in small spots and give the cottage cheesy look to the thighs, buttocks, arms, etc. Other experts believe the fat cells fill at different consistencies and create that lovely dimpling we all have learned to live with by covering up with wraps, shorts, skirts, etc. while we joyfully frolic on the beach. We really don't have a firm (no pun intended) answer as to what cellulite is and no one seems to be able to really define it in terms all experts will accept[4]. So, until we can decide what the heck it is, we treat it with modalities we hope and pray will work.

Endermologie is one of the devices used to treat cellulite. The FDA has approved these devices for the temporary reduction in the appearance of cellulite. Some newer devices use radio frequency to add a heated component that claims to heat up the fat, soften it, and lead to smoother skin. The procedure consists of the use of a hand piece by the technician to rub or knead the skin in certain spots of your body where the cellulite accumulates. You my, dear, are lying comfortably on a nice massage table wearing a body stocking and getting a treatment that feels like a very deep massage: Some say it's almost painful.

Your skin is basically vacuumed up in between the two rollers and the technician rolls it around the area for about 30 – 45 minutes. Some patients report bruising and swelling but hey, if the cellulite is gone, who cares? Both the device companies and providers suggest a minimum of 14 treatments spaced a few days apart at a price of $80 - $140 per treatment. This ranges from $1,120 to $1,960 for a series of sessions depending on the area of the body. Some initial swelling and redness is common. Again, you should know the results are temporary and it is recommended to receive monthly follow-up treatments.

Mesotherapy and Lipo-dissolve

Let's move on to the next cellulite "treatment". Well, actually, mesotherapy and lipo-dissolve claim to get rid of cellulite *and* reduce the size of an area. In other words, shrink thighs, hips, buttocks, belly, etc. with a simple injection! How marvelous... This treatment involves a series of multiple injections placed into an area that is deemed to have unsightly cellulite or bulges and then viola - it shrinks like magic! You just feel like you rolled onto a cactus but other than that, it's all-good. Oh, then there's the bruising and swelling that lasts for about two to four weeks on some people but there are reports of the swelling lasting much longer, months to years after treatment. Usually, after a few weeks it'll be time for your next treatment – ouch! How many times do you have to endure this torture? On average, about six. Yay.

The theory behind mesotherapy and lipo-dissolve is the patient is injected where there is an accumulation of fat, let's say the outer upper thigh. Anywhere from 10 to 40 sites are injected with a variety of combinations of medications, plant extracts, homeopathic substances, and/or vitamins. The mixture is supposed to target the fat cells and cause them to burst leading to the expulsion of their contents into the lymphatic system where it is drained away through the urine.

Clinicians that perform this have their own favorite mix or *cocktail* according to their unique protocol or according to how they were taught. There are many different combinations of many different substances but lipo-dissolve had its own specific mixture combination that was *secret* and only those clinicians who attended their trainings learned the magic potion's ingredients.

The FDA has not approved this method and also has taken steps to stop its use in the U.S[5]. As of this writing, some medical associations have issued health warnings regarding the use of mesotherapy and/or lipo-dissolve including the American Society of Plastic Surgeons, American Society for Aesthetic Plastic Surgery, and among others[6,7]. Additionally, the FDA has received reports of permanent scarring, painful knots under the skin, and skin deformity from the use of this type of therapy[8].

It is so disappointing that no one has come up with a safe, effective "cure" for cellulite. But, they haven't "cured" baldness either so I guess we'll have to put up with (and continue to love) our bald men and lumpy women for the time being... Let's face it, we all want smooth, cellulite-free skin and bodies but these treatments may not be the answer.

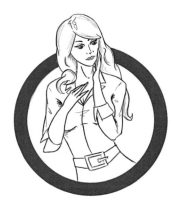

Chapter 9

WORKING WITH PLASTIC: COMBINING SURGICAL PROCEDURES WITH NON-SURGICAL TREATMENTS

Nip/Tuck

Ok, not everyone will be able to get by without surgery. Maybe just a little bit of a nip or tuck will do the trick. There are some things we just cannot correct with a needle or laser, for instance, those puffy little bags under the eyes, the tiny bit of excess skin on the upper lids, the face that has dropped a bit from all those birthdays in the sun. Aging is going to happen to all of us. It would be nice to do it slowly and gracefully so no one really knows what we've done, we just look better.

Where we may run into problems is waiting too long and not doing little bits along the way. For example, we all know someone who went from saggy skin and jowls to yanked tight overnight. Some unfortunate people are pulled so tightly, they can't close their eyes properly. That is a real shame because what we really want is to slow down the aging process and look our best. If non-surgical procedures, such as some of the treatments described in this book are done periodically, when/if it is time for the facelift or other procedure, it won't look odd or dramatic. The results will be soft and natural looking. Lots of plastic surgeons love working with aesthetic practitioners because together, we can create a pretty, natural, youthful look without going to extremes of either aspect.

The remainder of this chapter is written by a board certified plastic surgeon since they would be the experts in cosmetic surgery. Just in case you're wondering, yes, he's been on TV, yes, he worked in Beverly Hills, and yes, he is very talented. He currently has a practice in Newport Beach.

(I do not get any kickbacks from him. I've only done my research!)

Please meet Dr. Robert W. Kessler, M.D.
<u>Common Combinations of Surgical and Nonsurgical Techniques</u>

The traditional surgical mentality until about ten years ago was "nothing heals like cold steel", meaning anything of value was accomplished with a scalpel.

Current understanding of the aging process has changed all that, at least for those of us who pay attention.

The face ages in three characteristic ways. Classically we thought all aging was vertical which is why the surgical correction is called a "lift". Now we understand that in addition to this descent we experience volume loss. This is the reason for the growth of the filler industry and the use of fat transfer to refill the lost volume. Lastly we appreciate the loss of elasticity, color change and texture of the skin. Without addressing all three of these factors a total rejuvenation cannot be achieved.

Armed with this knowledge the approach to the face has been modified to address the underlying causes. There are now a number of surgical approaches that incorporate nonsurgical interventions to yield the desired aesthetic results.

When evaluating a person for facial rejuvenation, I always ask to see photos of them when they were younger. The goal is to restore their youthful appearance not to simply apply a technique that tightens the skin or raises the brows making them look like someone who has never walked the planet. These photos will guide the treatment and dictate the approach needed to achieve our desires.

In consultation for facial rejuvenation I begin at the forehead and work my way down to the neck evaluating each area. Treatment options are reviewed with the patient in a particular region of the face beginning with non-surgical techniques and progressing to surgical options if necessary. By the end of the consultation it is clear what the best options are and you will decide which plan is best for you. This is important because you should be very involved in the decisions affecting your face.

When evaluating the brow it is important to measure the distance from the eyebrow to the hairline, note the position of the inner aspect of the brow relative to the outer aspect and if the hair of the eyebrow is actually below the bony orbital rim; it is not just the arch form that is critical in this decision making process. The brows can be lifted chemically with Botox, endoscopically (a small, flexible tube) using small incisions in the hairline, or with an open technique that can reduce the length of the forehead and advance the hairline.

Upper eyelid evaluation must always include assessment of the brow. Often a low brow is a more significant contributor to the appearance of the upper lid than the upper lid skin itself. The upper lids can do very nicely with laser resurfacing alone if the excess is mild to moderate. The fractional CO_2 lasers as discussed previously do a great job of tightening and smoothing the skin on these patients. Skin excision and fat removal is often necessary when the upper lids appear full and this can only be addressed surgically.

Lower eyelids have been a challenge for surgeons as the volume loss in the tear trough area below the bony rim exaggerates the fullness of the lower lid. In addition to volume loss of the lower lid there is weakening of the muscles in this area, which create the characteristic "bags" we see as we age. Surgical removal of the skin and fat helps the appearance of the area but does not restore collagen to the skin that remains. The eyelid skin is the thinnest skin in the body and the underlying muscle shows through this thin skin and makes the area appear dark. Products that hydrate the skin diffuse the light making this darkness less perceptible. Laser thickens the skin over the muscle and improves the skin quality, and in addition to smoothing out fine lines it diminishes those dreaded dark circles as well. Surgically, we have the ability to remove the fat and skin, repositioning the fat into the tear trough and tear trough implants also address this issue nicely. Surgical removal of the lower lid fat through an incision on the inside of the eyelid can be performed along with laser resurfacing of the eyelids with a wonderful improvement and no visible scars. But now with the use of Restylane the transition between the cheek and lower lid can be greatly improved non-surgically in the office. By replacing volume in the tear trough the transition from lower lid fullness to the cheek is blended restoring the youthful appearance of the eye. The skin of the lower lid responds beautifully to laser resurfacing and often the combination of volume replacement and laser is the solution to a youthful lower lid. The advent of fillers has made a great contribution to the lower lid aesthetics.

Endoscopic surgical techniques, use of a camera and instruments placed through small openings in the skin, have also made significant improvements to the surgical approach to the face and body. Generally speaking if a less invasive technique is used, additional procedures can be done at the same time. The endoscope can be used to lift the forehead and the face making this minimal access surgery easily combined with laser and fat transfer in one procedure. This is possible because there is less manipulation of tissue that interferes with blood supply, and can lead to wound healing problems.

The traditional facelift remains the gold standard for *surgical* facial rejuvenation but it has been improved by the addition of facial fillers, fat transfer and finally fractional laser resurfacing of the skin when necessary. The volume augmentation can be done during surgery with fat transfer from the tummy or love handles or it can be done after surgery with many of the fine fillers that you have learned about earlier in this book. The facelift will place structures back in their appropriate positions while the volume can be restored to its more youthful state. Once the structure and volume are set the 'veneer' of the face must be addressed. Light based treatments like

IPL and fractional laser can help with pigmentation and fine lines. These techniques are usually performed after the facelift due to healing concerns at the time of the surgery.

Finally, understand that not all practitioners have the same level of experience or artistic insights. Cosmetic surgery is a unique field in medicine. It is the only medical field, where we operate on perfectly healthy people for the sole purpose of making them look better. Removing an appendix in New York is done exactly the same way as it is in Newport Beach but listen to three consultations with Board Certified Plastic surgeons and I assure you they will each have different approaches and different aesthetic outcomes. Seek out experienced Board Certified Plastic and Facial Plastic surgeons and make sure you feel comfortable with who you choose to perform your procedure. I strongly recommend you look at before and after photos of work done by your surgeon to confirm that you share their aesthetic sense and will be getting the results you desire. This can be a wonderfully transformative experience but you need to do your homework, it is *your face* after all.

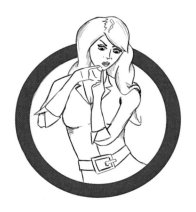

Chapter 10

ACNE - PIMPLES AT MY AGE?

Are you kidding me?

There are more than a few words that can describe the feeling we get when we get one or more pimples on our face; distressing, embarrassed, mad, concerned, obsessed, the list of adjectives goes on and on. When we are teenagers we kind of expect a pimple or two or ten but that doesn't mean it's fun. You are considered to have acne if you have one or more raised open comedones (black-heads) or pustules (pimple or white-heads) on your face or body. Common areas affected by acne are the face, the back, the chest, and the shoulders because the sebaceous glands are the largest in these areas[1]. A few unfortunate people suffer with acne on their abdomen as well.

Some teens have a significant problem with acne causing scarring that lasts into their later years and is often permanent. Additionally, many people in their 40's and 50's *start* getting acne and are completely blindsided because they've "never had a pimple in their life!" According to a survey of over 1000 adults, self-reported acne was documented for men and women as:

- 20 to 29 years: 43 and 51 percent, respectively
- 30 to 39 years: 20 and 35 percent, respectively
- 40 to 49 years: 12 and 26 percent, respectively
- 50 and older: 7 and 15 percent, respectively[2]

The above list shows that more women than men complain of adult onset acne.

This portion of the book will offer insight to and remedies for acne, a fascinating but frustrating condition.

What is Acne?

Acne is a condition that results in the formation of pustules and blackheads from some disruption in the skin, specifically the pilosebaceous unit or the area where the oil glands and hair follicles reside[3]. It is not fully understood but basically what happens is the skin cells that line the follicle shed and become a little sticky before they get outside of the follicle. They become sticky from getting "old" in the follicle from trying to shed, but they are being held back. They are getting blocked by other cells and then build up onto themselves.

Since they are sticky, they clump and cause an inflammatory response underneath the skin surface. This inflammatory response causes the redness, swelling and debris (white cells that make the whitehead) to accumulate inside the follicle and voila – you have an acne lesion[4]. Sometimes there are little open comedones that contain puddles of those sticky cells that attract bacteria and provide a lovely home for them to multiply and cause havoc. Hence, another, different kind acne lesion is born, the blackhead. But wait, there's more.

When that bothersome white pustule rises to the surface of your skin, you probably whip out your mirror and squeeze the crap out of it. After a good amount of painful squeezing and injuring your skin, the goo comes out. Ah, when that white stuff comes popping out of your skin it's such a feeling of accomplishment – "I got it!" Unfortunately, there is a down side to doing this to your face. First of all, you are causing post-traumatic hyperpigmentation, the red mark that stays as a reminder of your pimple for a few weeks to years. Additionally, when you squeeze that pimple, half of the pressure and debris shoots out of your skin but the other portion stays put and can even travel to different areas nearby and, you guessed it, cause another pimple. See, your mother was right when she told you not to pick at your face!

If you can't resist the temptation to pick at your face when you see a pesky white pustule, do not squeeze the pimple. Gently use a cotton swab to lightly push on the pimple from one side only. If the debris does not come out easily – STOP! You can try again in the morning. If it does come out, do not squeeze the pimple but let the debris drain out slowly. Then dab the pimple with one of the recommended products in the acne remedy section. This may help you avoid the red or brown marks and increased acne pimples in the future.

Now, you might be wondering why teenagers are so prone to acne. Well, their hormones (androgens) have a lot to do with it (mom was right again!) What happens to those poor, unsuspecting teenagers is their hormones cause the sebaceous gland to become very active, grow and secrete more and more sebum (oil)[5]. When there is an increase in oil production, there is an increased chance of the cells getting sticky and clogging the follicles. The reason some of the over the counter products containing benzoyl peroxide and/or salicylic acid work so well on acne lesions is because these products get into the follicle somewhat and help prevent the cells from sticking together.

Hormones continue to affect our skin into adulthood. Testosterone regulates the secretion of oil in men and the luteinizing hormone (LH) affects the oil production in women. There is a sharp increase in LH secretion after ovulation and this causes an increase in oil production that leads to acne about two to seven days before menstruation[6]. Now it's all making sense isn't it? The reason oral contraceptives containing estrogen improve acne is because it suppresses ovarian production of testosterone (yes women make testosterone too) and provides a more steady state of hormones. Testosterone plays a significant role in oil production[7].

Another variation of acne is called acne mechanica. This may cause acne through mechanical disruption or blockage of the pilosebaceous unit through pressure from such things as helmets, hats, turtleneck sweaters, phones, resting the head or face on the hand(s), and other causes producing even a slight amount of pressure[8]. Take a look in the mirror and see if you notice more acne on one side or the other. Think back. Did you used to rest your cheek in your hand during class or while reading a book? Or do you use your cell phone on the acne-affected side? It might be worth changing some habits that could be causing breakouts in that area.

Topical Products That May Cause Acne-type Breakouts

People often use products that contain ingredients that make their skin feel softer and smoother, especially on the face. If there are certain products you use that cause your skin to breakout, look at the ingredients. You may have what's called acne cosmetica (i.e. acne type breakouts from certain cosmetic ingredients). Or another variation called acne pomade, get it? This one is from hair products (pomade) and commonly affects the forehead[9].

Some of the common ingredients that incite acne are:

1. Mineral oil

2. Lanolin

3. Coconut oils

4. Wax, beeswax

5. Heavy oil based hair products

Be aware though, sometimes it's not the product but how you apply or use it. If you are vigorously scrubbing, rubbing or massaging your skin when you use the suspicious product, it may not be the ingredient but how you are using it instead[10]. Yes, you need to practically become a detective.

Diet Related to Acne

There is no conclusive evidence that diet has anything to do with acne. However, there have been some studies suggesting there is a link between acne and consuming milk. Diets that included milk consumption of more than three servings a week appeared to be associated with an increase in acne[11]. These studies were not conclusive but did suggest some relationship. If you or a loved one is desperate, you can surely try giving up milk for a couple of months and see what happens. Fingers crossed.

Are you ready for some great news? "There is no reliable evidence that ingesting chocolate is associated with an increased prevalence or severity of acne"[12]. Hip-hip hooray! Pass the Godiva please...

Other than that, there is not much in the way of diet affecting acne so no need to worry about that. Now you can concentrate on things that are really going to help.

Acne in Women

Acne in women is caused by the same factors listed previously; excess oil production through hormones, bacteria, sticky cells, and inflammation. Unique to women is a condition known as polycystic ovarian syndrome where the ovaries produce increased amounts of androgens and can cause acne through complicated mechanisms[13]. A visit with your primary or women's health care clinician is a great way to get an evaluation.

Another aspect unique to women suffering with acne is, fluctuating hormones during the menstrual cycle. As previously discussed, hormones cause more oil production and therefore increase the number of acne lesions. Women may benefit from oral hormonal contraceptives in the treatment of their acne. Of course, pregnancy should be discussed as well as future family planning when being treated for acne with any type of medication.

Acne Remedies

Although it's hard to tell which products in skin care and cosmetic products will clog pores, and the importance of cosmetic products as contributors to acne is uncertain, many experts recommend the use of skin care products (eg, moisturizers, cleansers, cosmetics, etc.) labeled as "non-comedogenic" and "non-acnegenic" for people with acne. In addition, if you like to use foundation as part of your makeup routine, select "oil-free" liquid silicone (dimethicone or cyclomethicone) matte foundations over oil-containing products, because the silicone-based products may be less clogging[14].

One commonly recommended acne prevention regimen follows:

- In the morning, cleanse with a salicylic acid facial wash, apply a topical antibiotic or azelaic acid (both prescription), and of course a sunscreen. If the skin is oily, there are "drier" sunscreens available over the counter as well as some powder sunscreens as previously mentioned in the skin care chapter. In the evening, cleanse with the same cleanser as used in the morning and then apply a topical retinoid (prescription). This regimen can certainly be tailored to fit the patient's needs and can be determined by the clinician.

The following table describes the five treatments steps for acne as outlined by Baumann (2002)[15].

Step 1: Preventing skin cells from sticking together

Step 2: Eliminating or reducing bacteria

Step 3: Removing the debris that clogs pores

Step 4: Attacking the inflammatory response

Step 5: Decrease the level of sebum (oil)

Prevention of sticky cells	Eliminate bacteria	Remove debris that clogs pores	Attack the inflammation	Decrease the amount of oil
Retinoids	Topical antibiotic creams/gels	Retinoids	Salicylic acid wash (over the counter)	Oral contraceptives
Accutane	Benzoyl peroxide preparations	Salicylic acid	In-office peels	Retinoids
Tazorac	Azelaic acid	Glycolic acid	Oral anti-inflammatory (ibuprofen, naproxen, etc.)	
Differin	Oral antibiotics	Lactic acid		
		Azelaic acid		

As you can see, retinoids are used in several steps and are considered the 'gold standard' by many experts today for treatment of acne[16]. The problem with retinoids is they can cause some redness, drying, flaking, and irritation of the skin. These are the reasons that teens don't continue using this medication even though it may be very effective.

Other remedies for acne that work well are IPL treatments, photodynamic therapy (PDT) with levulinic acid, and commercialized acne regimens that include the active ingredients listed above. Teens have an easier time with treatments that are simple to use and effective in a short amount of time, they are just too impatient. Photodynamic therapy is an excellent choice for teens (or anyone for that matter) that want speedy results without the step-by-step regimens of other acne treatments. A thorough consultation with an experienced clinician is strongly recommended to determine if the PDT is an option since there is a light-based component to it. In-office peels are another good choice for control of acne. Most people need a combination of office based treatments and home regimens to get the best results.

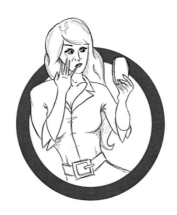

Chapter 11

WHAT HAPPENED TO MY BEAUTIFUL SKIN? MATURE SKIN.

The Golden Age

Getting older causes changes in our skin. Just because we've accumulated more birthdays than our friends or neighbors doesn't mean we have to "give up" or "give in" to looking older. As we age, our skin goes through a transformation of sorts that is different than sun damage. Sun damage is addressed in previous chapters along with specific improvement options for specific concerns. Aging skin changes, regardless of sun exposure, and includes the following properties; dryness, loosening/sagging of the skin, broken capillaries, thinning, and slower shedding of dead skin cells. There is also a 50 percent overall reduction in nail growth and reductions in sweat and sebaceous gland activity, so no wonder the skin feels dry[1].

Additional changes associated with aging in both men and women, rather than sun damage, include the following:

- The dermis thins with a decrease in vascularity that contributes to delayed wound healing.

- The elastic fiber network degenerates significantly after we hit 40 years old because we do not produce the same amount of elastin as we did when we were younger and this leads to loss of hydration and decreased skin resilience.

- The ability to deliver heat to the skin for excretion is impaired and that's why older people tend to complain of being cold. The natural loss of sub-dermal fat decreases insulation and the ability of older people to conserve heat. Decreases in both number and production of sweat glands, also contribute to impaired thermoregulation with aging[2].

Topical administration of retinoids appears to reverse many of the age-related changes in sun-protected skin. After approximately nine months of daily treatment with topical retinoid cream, the epidermis thickened, capillaries reappeared, and collagen and elastin increased. Thus, these age-related changes appear to be amenable to improvement[3].

Aging for women is a little different than that for men. Our skin tends to be thinner than men's skin and seems to collect fine lines more easily. Further, many women report unwelcomed changes in their hair, nails and skin with the onset of menopause – how fun ☹.

Estrogen influences skin thickness so decreasing levels of estrogen in both surgical (total hysterectomy) and natural menopausal women, cause the skin to become thinner, less elastic and more susceptible to cuts and bruises[4].

Declining levels of estrogen also leads to increased levels of testosterone floating around so then we may also get to enjoy increased facial hair – marvelous! And remember, lasers don't work for hair reduction on gray hair. More mature women with gray facial hair will have to tweeze, thread, or get electrolysis treatments. On top of that, decreased estrogen also causes the hair from the scalp to shed in such a way that it appears thinner. Most of the time this scalp shedding will level out and there is no therapy for it so take care of the hair you have[5].

Unfortunately, there isn't a whole lot we can do about the skin changes caused from menopause. Menopausal levels of estrogen leave us with few choices other than use hormonal replacement therapy but that is an individual decision made between you and your health care provider based on your personal health history, family history, lifestyle, and other factors.

Some options women might do for their skin are; to get regular facials and microdermabrasions. These treatments help your skin look its best and also allows the aesthetician to recommend products for your skin type that best suits you and your needs. Sometimes night creams work well during the daytime on women that have very dry skin. Just because the label says "night cream" don't be afraid to use it during the day. Night creams tend to have more emollients and moisturizing ingredients than the lighter daytime creams or lotions.

There are different preparations of products for use on the face like creams, lotions, gels, and serums. *Creams* are the "heaviest" of the moisturizing preparations and also provide a barrier so the water in the skin does not evaporate as quickly. *Lotions* are lighter, absorb a bit more, and do not sit on top of the skin as much as creams; lotions are good choices for people with oily/combination skin. *Gels* absorb quickly into the skin and often need additional moisturizer. Further, if you are using a *serum* for rejuvenation that contains active ingredients such as vitamin C or kojic acid, you'll need to use a lotion or cream on top of that for moisture. Serums are usually comprised of active ingredients that are absorbed quickly into the skin and are not very moisturizing. So, for more mature, drier skin, serums using active ingredients for rejuvenation (see the chapter on skin care) in combination with a moisturizing cream would be a good start. More mature skin also responds wonderfully to the fractional laser treatments as these treatments thicken the skin through collagen production.

Realizing the skin will lose its elasticity and resilience can at least alert you to take care of the skin you have. Drink plenty of water to stay hydrated, keep your skin moisturized, and avoid prolonged sun exposure at all costs! Our skin is going to age anyway so we certainly do not want to speed up the break down and aging process of our skin. Our skin has been working all its life to protect us, fight off invaders, heat us, cool us, and help us look "put together". You owe it to yourself to take good care of the largest organ of your body.

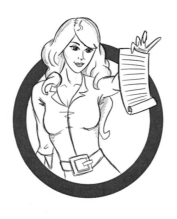

Chapter 12

PATIENT TESTIMONIALS

Why we do what we do

Have you thought about why you'd like to get medical cosmetic treatments done? Have you ever wondered why your friends have chosen to get treatments and what helped them make their decision? Well, here are some answers (of course you can ask your friends yourself). There are of course other opinions but below are the majority of responses WHY people explore aesthetic treatment options.

According to a study by Maley (2007), the number one reason (39%) people decided to get a medical cosmetic procedure was to look younger. Next was to look better (38%), then to find romance (11%), then recently divorced and wanted a change (6%), finally had the money (4%), and the remaining 2% included; stay competitive, saw a friend's result and wanted the same, special occasion, fight aging process, and felt better when better looking. Some actual quotes from Maley's study are:

"I don't mind getting older but I do mind looking old"

"I want to turn back the clock"

"I will fight this aging process to the end!"

"I want to look in the mirror and feel good about what I see"

"I'm proud of staying in great shape and want my face to reflect my body"

"I feel more confident when I look good"

As you can tell by these comments, people want to look their best, not over done and unusual. This applies to both men and women. Millions of men and women receive cosmetic treatments every year and the majority of them visit their aesthetic clinician several times a year for different treatments and suggestions. Here is what some of my patients are saying:

"I'm not sure why I waited so long to get Botox. I think I was nervous about how it would look since I've heard stories and also saw a movie where the guy had crazy eyebrows. Also, I wasn't thrilled about having needles in my face. Well, now I

know! It is a super easy, painless treatment and I LOVE the results! I look refreshed and lifted - I can't believe I waited so long!" **Monica 47, aesthetic patient of 7 years.**

"Who on Earth discovered [fillers]! What a genius! I am so glad I don't have to get a facelift for many years since I get my cheeks done with Perlane. That stuff gives my face a lift and makes me look years younger but doesn't make me look like someone else! I love it so much and if I wasn't so vain, I'd tell everyone what I do to look this good..." **Susan 50, aesthetic patient of 5 years**

"Three words - I love Dysport" **Henry, 42, aesthetic patient of 2 years**

"Of course I want to look my best, I am in real estate. So I indulge in these treatments. Shhh, it's a secret but I get regular microdermabrasions, Botox, and IPL. What a difference! I think I sell more homes because I look fresh - Haha!" **Paula, 39, aesthetic patient of 4 years**

" I have struggled with acne since I was a kid. Now I'm 23 and still have occasional breakouts but since using products and treatments recommended by my [practitioner (Beth)], I have much clearer skin and only random pimples. Chemical peels are also great before I go back to school and keep my skin in better condition for a couple of months" **Sara, 23, aesthetic patient of 8 years**

If you have been curious lately about certain procedures or products you can start doing some research and find an office you like, maybe through a friend or another recommendation. But, after reading this book you should be armed with enough knowledge to make informed decisions to get the results you want! You can easily make an appointment for a consultation – there should be zero pressure to get anything done at that appointment unless YOU decide you want to move forward right then and there (which happens a lot). Just because you filled out a form or two and signed a consent form, doesn't mean anyone will touch you, you are in control. And, the consultations are *usually* no charge but on occasion, if you schedule with a plastic surgeon there might be a fee. In many cases, it will be credited towards any procedure you may have.

Cosmetic treatments can be as easy as a microdermabrasion or a facial that you get once a month to a fractional CO_2 laser resurfacing that you may get once every 5 - 10 years, or a combination of different treatments. It's all up to you and what you are comfortable with, financially, emotionally, and physically.

You don't have to undergo surgery to get amazing results but you will likely have to endure some type of sacrifice like time, money, or maybe even a temporary bruise. Don't be scared, for most people it's very much worth it and you will literally be wondering why you waited so long. Welcome to the Club!

Before & After Treatment Photos

IPL Facial Treatments

BEFORE   **AFTER**

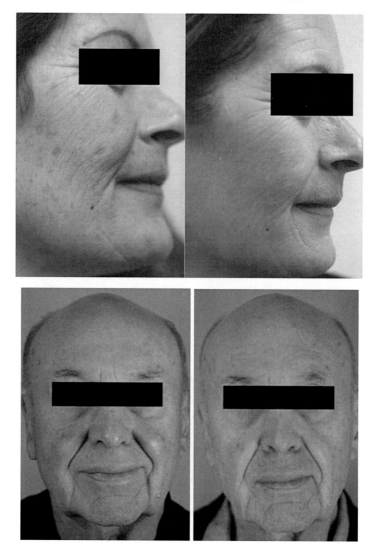

<u>IPL Hand Treatments</u>

BEFORE

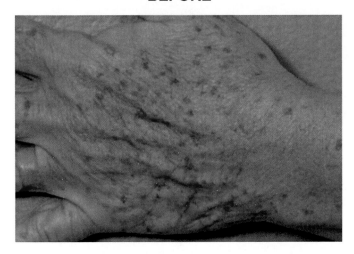

AFTER

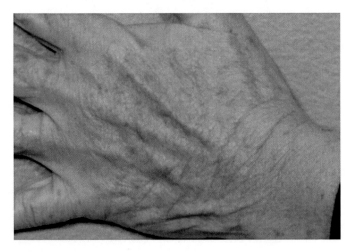

Filler Treatments

<u>Lips & Naso-labial folds</u>

BEFORE

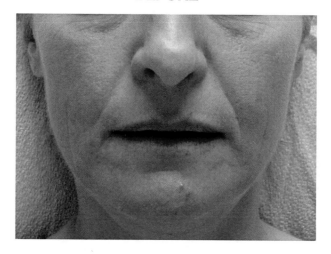

2 DAYS AFTER

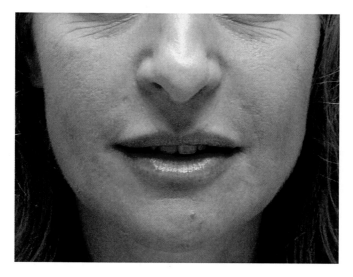

<u>Lips & Naso-labial folds (Con't)</u>

BEFORE

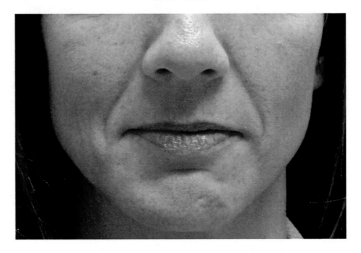

AFTER

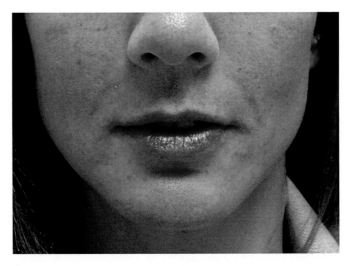

<u>Cheeks</u>

BEFORE

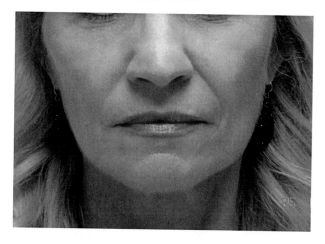

AFTER

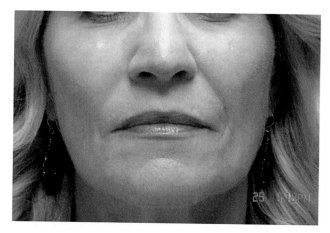

<u>Cheeks & Lips</u>

BEFORE

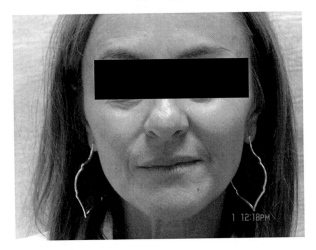

AFTER

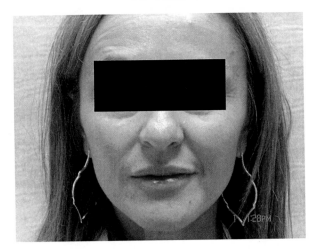

Appendix

Also Known As (aka) and Pricing

First, let's look at the most common names associated with the more popular treatments and procedures. Depending on the state, region, county, city or town you live in or visit for your aesthetic treatments, some treatments and procedures will be called something different. The commonly used name will be listed first and the aka will be in the table after the name. In some cases, there will not be an aka so the box will be left blank.

Intense Pulsed Light (IPL)	IPL, photofacial, photo-facial, foto-facial, light facial
Laser Hair Removal (LHR)	Laser hair reduction
Lower Face Lift	Diamond lift, lite-lift, lunch-time lift, others
Upper/Lower Blephroplasty	Upper eyelid surgery, lid job, under eye bag removal
Augmentation with filler (Cheeks, temples, chin, jawline, eyebrows, lips and other areas of the face).	Liquid face-lift, liquid lift, facial rejuvenation, lip plumping, facial contouring, lip enhancement, vampire lift

CO2 laser resurfacing	Laser peel, laser rejuvenation, Fraxel, DOT, Madonna lift
Sclerotherapy	Vein treatment, vein injections
Botox, Dysport	Wrinkle treatment

Pricing

Pricing can be all over the map. Following is a price range of the most common prices. You'll have to do a little investigating on your own for your particular area. It is recommended you do not shop for lowest price, rather shop for best quality. Also consider how you feel if you make an appointment for a consultation. Are you uncomfortable? Pushed? Rushed? Feel like you're being sold the farm? Or do you feel comfortable, welcome, and safe?

Laser hair reduction – $50 – 4500 depending on area of the body and if charged per session or per package of 5 sessions

IPL (face) – $99 – 400, other areas of the body i.e. neck, chest, hands, arms vary widely in price.

Botox – per unit $8 - 20, per area $100 – 400 Typical usage is approximately 30 – 60 units. (Some offices charge by the unit of Botox/Dysport and customize the treatment to your unique face and musculature whereas others charge by the area treated i.e. forehead is a flat fee no matter how much or little used).

Dysport – per unit: $3 - 5, per area: $100 – 400. Typical usage is 50 – 150 units.

CO2 fractional laser resurfacing - $350 – 6,000 per treatment, depending on area of the face/body

Microdermabrasion - $80 – 150 per treatment

Dermal fillers (Restylane, Perlane, Juvederm) - $350 – 700 per 1 mL syringe. Typical use: 1 mL for lips, 2 – 4 mL for cheeks, 1 – 3 mL for naso-labial folds (smile lines)

Sculptra – $800 – 4000. Depending on number of treatments.

Radiesse – $600 - 2000

Photodynamic therapy - $400 – 1000 per treatment, more than one may be necessary.

In-office chemical Peels - $100 – 500

**Surgical options vary widely and a consultation is recommended where you will decide with the surgeon your best options and pricing.

Sources

CHAPTER 1
1. http://www.merriam-webster.com/dictionary/perfectionist
2. American Society of Plastic Surgeons (2012). Retrieved from: http://www.plasticsurgery.org/Documents/news-resources/statistics/2011-statistics/2011_Stats_Quick_Facts.pdf
3. WebMD (2012). History of make-up. Retrieved from: http://www.webmd.com/healthybeauty/guide/history-makeup
4. Centers for disease control and prevention (CDC, 2012). Retrieved from http://www.cdc.gov/healthyweight/assessing/bmi/adult_bmi/index.html
5. Robbins, J (1998) *Diet for a new America: How your food choices affect your health, happiness, and the future of life on earth.* Stillpoint Publisher: CA.
6. Chao, A, Thun, M.J., Connell, C.J., McCullough, M.L., Jacobs, E.J., Flanders, W.D., et al. (2005). Meat consumption and risk of colorectal cancer. *Journal of the American Medical Association 293*, (2).
7. Boeker, et al. (2008). The runner's high: Opioidergic mechanisms in the human brain. Cerebral Cortex: Oxford University Press doi:10.1093/cercor/bhn013
8. Botox cosmetic: OnabotulinumtoxinA (2011) Allergan Inc. Retrieved from: http://www.allergan.com/assets/pdf/botox_cosmetic/pi.pdf

CHAPTER 2

1. Kolarsick, P.A., Kolarsick, M.A., & Goodwin, C. (2011). Anatomy and physiology of the skin. *Journal of the dermatology nurses association,* vol 3, (4).
2. Ibid, 207-208.
3. Ibid, 208.
4. Paus, R. & Cotsarelis, G. (1999). The biology of hair follicles. New England journal of Medicine; vol. 341 (7).
5. Kolarsick, P.A., Kolarsick, M.A., & Goodwin, C. (2011). Anatomy and physiology of the skin. *Journal of the dermatology nurses association,* vol 3, (4).
6. Ibid, 210.
7. Seeley, R.R., Stephens, T.D., & Tate, P. (1989). *Anatomy and physiology.* St. Louis, MI: Times Mirror/Mosby College Publishing.
8. Ibid, 678.
9. Ibid, 117.
10. Baumann, L. (2002). Cosmetic Dermatology: Principals and practice. McGraw-Hill, NY.
11. Ibid, 79
12. Brice,S. & Shift, K.R. (2012). Sunburn. *Up To Date.* Retrieved from: http://www.uptodate.com/contents/sunburn
13. U.S. Department of Health and Human Services, Public Health Service, National Toxicology Program, (2011). *Report on carcinogens, eleventh edition (ultraviolet radiation related exposures).* Retrieved from: http://ntp.niehs.nih.gov/index.cfm?objectid=B E5743A8-F1F6-975E-788AFA05237BE33C

14. D'Souza, G. & Evans, G. (2007). Mexoryl: A review of an ultraviolet A Filter. *Plastic and reconstructive surgery, 120* (4). Retrieved from: http://journals.lww.com/plasreconsurg/Abstrac t/2007/09150/Mexoryl__A_Review_of_an_Ul traviolet_A_Filter.33.aspx doi: 10.1097/01.prs.0000280561.02915.3a

15. US Food and drug administration (2012). Questions and Answers: FDA announces new requirements for over-the-counter (OTC) sunscreen products marketed in the U.S. Retrieved from: http://www.fda.gov/Drugs/ResourcesForYou/ Consumers/BuyingUsingMedicineSafely/Und erstandingOver-the-CounterMedicines/ucm258468.htm

16. Sun & Skin News (2011). FDA issues new sunscreen labeling rules. Vol. 28, (2). The Skin Cancer Foundation: New York

17. Baumann, L. (2002). Cosmetic Dermatology: Principals and practice. McGraw-Hill, NY.

18. Up-to-Date (2011). Hydroquinone Drug information; Lexicomp. Retrieved from: www.uptodate.com

19. Garcia, A. & Fulton, J.E. (1996). The combination of glycolic acid and hydroquinone or kojic acid for the treatment of melisma or related conditions. *Dermatological Surgery*: 22, pp. 443-447

20. Up-to-Date (2011). Topical tretinoin (topical all trans retinoic acid): Drug information; Lexicomp. Retrieved from: www.uptodate.com

21. Ibid.

22. Food and drug administration (2011). Classification of Products as Drugs and Devices and Additional Product Classification Issues. Retrieved from: http://www.fda.gov/RegulatoryInformation/G uidances/ucm258946.htm#_Toc294261434

23. Food and Drug Administration (2011). Is It a Cosmetic, a Drug, or Both? (Or Is It Soap?). Retrieved from: http://www.fda.gov/Cosmetics/GuidanceCom plianceRegulatoryInformation/ucm074201.ht m

24. Ibid.

25. Graf, J. (2010). Antioxidants and skin care: the Essentials. *Plastic and reconstructive surgery*, 125 (1).

26. Ibid, 379-381.

27. Ibid, 379.

28. Baxter, R.A. (2008). Anti-aging properties of resveratrol: review and report of a potent new antioxidant skin care formulation. *Journal of cosmetic dermatology*, 7.

29. Baumann, L. (2007). Less known botanical cosmeceuticals. *Dermatologic therapy*, (20). Blackwell publishing.

30. Graf, J. (2010). Antioxidants and skin care: the Essentials. *Plastic and reconstructive surgery*, 125 (1).

31. Baumann, L. (2007). Less known botanical cosmeceuticals. *Dermatologic therapy,*(20). Blackwell publishing.

32. Graf, J. (2010). Antioxidants and skin care: the Essentials. *Plastic and reconstructive surgery*, 125 (1).

33. Kneedler, J.A., Sexton, L.R., & Sky, S.S. (1998). Understanding alpha hydroxyl acids. *Dermatology nursing,*(10), 4.

34. Baumann, L. (2002). Cosmetic Dermatology: Principals and practice. McGraw-Hill, NY.

35. Ibid, 111 – 112.

36. Graf, J. (2010). Antioxidants and skin care: the Essentials. *Plastic and reconstructive surgery*, 125 (1).

37. Baumann, L. (2002). Cosmetic Dermatology: Principals and practice. McGraw-Hill, NY.

38. Ibid, 101 – 102.

39. University of Maryland Medical Center, (2011) Coenzyme Q 10. Retrieved from http://www.umm.edu/altmed/articles/coenzym e-q10-000295.htm

40. Graf, J. (2010). Antioxidants and skin care: the Essentials. *Plastic and reconstructive surgery*, 125 (1).

41. Garcia, A. & Fulton, J.E. (1996). The combination of glycolic acid and hydroquinone or kojic acid for the treatment

of melisma or related conditions. Dermatological Surgery: 22, pp. 443-447

42. Lambert, C. (2005). Deep into sleep. *Harvard magazine.*

CHAPTER 3
1. American society of plastic surgeons (2012). Retrieved from: http://www.plasticsurgery.org/cosmetic-procedures/microdermabrasion.html
2. Ibid.
3. American society of plastic surgeons (2012). Retrieved from: http://www.plasticsurgery.org/cosmetic-procedures/dermabrasion.html?sub=Dermabra sion%20procedural%20steps
4. American society of plastic surgeons (2012). Retrieved from: http://www.plasticsurgery.org/cosmetic-procedures/chemical-peel
5. Ibid.
6. Ibid.
7. Ibid.
8. Latisse prescribing highlights (2012). Retrieved from: http://www.allergan.com/assets/pdf/latisse_pi.pdf
9. Ibid.

CHAPTER 4

1. Mann, M.W., Berk, D.R., Popkin, D.L., & Bayliss, S.J. (2011). *Handbook of Dermatology: a Practical manual.* Blackwell publishing.

2. Encyclopedia of Laser Physics and Technology: A - M, Volume 1 (2008). By Rüdiger Paschotta pp. 160, 370, 377-8 Wiley-VCH

3. Hruza, G.J., J. S., Dover, & Ofori, A. O. 2012 April. Principles of lasers and intense pulsed light for cutaneous lesions. *UpToDate.com* Retrieved from: http://www.uptodate.com/contents/principles-of-laser-and-intense-pulsed-light-for-cutaneouslesions?source=search_result&search=photorejuvenation&selectedTitle=1%7E1#H1638085

4. Ibid.

5. Hsu, T. & Kaminer, M.S. (2003). The use of nonablative radiofrequency technology to tighten the lower face and neck. *Seminars in cutaneous medicine and surgery 22* (2), pp. 115 – 123.

6. Bassichis, B.A., Dayan, S., & Thomas, J.R. (2004). Use of a nonablative radiofrequency device to rejuvenate the upper one-third of the face. *Otolaryngology - head and neck surgery 130* (4), pp.397 – 406.

7. Dover,J.S. & Zelickson, B. (2007). Results of a Survey of 5,700 Patient Monopolar

Radiofrequency Facial Skin Tightening Treatments: Assessment of a Low-Energy Multiple-Pass Technique Leading to a Clinical End Point Algorithm. *Dermatologic surgery 33* (8) pp. 900 - 907.

8. Finzi, E. & Spangler, A. (2005). Multipass Vector (Mpave) Technique with Nonablative Radiofrequency to Treat Facial and Neck Laxity. *Dermatological surgery31* (8), pp. 916-922.

CHAPTER 5

1. Botox cosmetic: OnabotulinumtoxinA (2011) Allergan Inc. retrieved from http://www.allergan.com/assets/pdf/botox_cos metic_pi.pdf

CHAPTER 6

1. Matarasso, S. L. & Beer, K. (2005). Injectable collagens. *Soft tissue augmentation* (pp.19 – 20). Philadelphia: Elsevier.
2. Food and drug administration (2009). *Restylane injectable gel.* Retrieved from: http://www.fda.gov/MedicalDevices
3. Ibid.
4. Lowe, N.J., Maxwell, A., Lowe, P., Duick, M.G., & Shah, K. (2001). Hyaluronic acid fillers: Adverse reactions and skin testing. *Journal of the American academy of dermatologists 44*, pp. 930-933.

152

5. American Society of Plastic Surgeons (2012). Retrieved from: http://www.plasticsurgery.org/Documents/new s-resources/statistics/2011-statistics/2011_Stats_Quick_Facts.pdf
6. Carruthers, J. & Carruthers, A. (2005) Procedures in dermatology: Soft tissue augmentation. Elsevier Saunders
7. Ibid, 98
8. Bowman, P.H, & Narins, R.S. (2005). Hylans and soft tissue augmentation. Soft tissue augmentation (pp. 33-41). Philadelphia: Elsevier.
9. Carruthers, J. & Carruthers, A. (2005) Procedures in dermatology: Soft tissue augmentation. Elsevier Saunders.

CHAPTER 7
1. Paschotta, R. (2008). Encyclopedia of Laser Physics and Technology: A - M, Volume 1, pp. 160, 370, 377-8 Wiley-VCH
2. Shenenberger, D.W. (2012). Removal of unwanted hair. Retrieved from: Up to Date http://www.uptodate.com/contents/removal-of-unwanted-hair
3. Ibid.
4. Paus, R. & Cotsarelis, G. (1999). The biology of hair follicles. *New England journal of Medicine, 341* (7).

5. Goldberg, D.J., Dover, J.S., & Ofori, A.O. (2012). Ablative laser resurfacing for skin rejuvenation. *UpToDate.com* Retrieved from: http://www.uptodate.com/contents/ablative-laser-resurfacing-for-skin-rejuvenation
6. Ibid.
7. Ibid.
8. Ibid.
9. Ibid.

CHAPTER 8

1. Nicholas, C., Elliot, L., Sharpe, C., & Sharpe, D. (1999). Cellulite Treatment: A Myth or Reality: A Prospective Randomized, Controlled Trial of Two Therapies, Endermologie and Aminophylline Cream. *Plastic & Reconstructive Surgery*: *104* (4) – pp. 1110-1114.
2. Baumann, L. (2002). Cosmetic Dermatology: Principals and practice. McGraw-Hill, NY.
3. Avram, M. M. (2004). Cellulite: a Review of its physiology and treatment. *Journal of cosmetic and laser therapy 6* (4) 181-185 doi: 10.1080/14764170410003057
4. Ibid.
5. Food and drug administration. *FDA information on lipodissolve* (2010). Retrieved from:

http://www.fda.gov/Drugs/GuidanceComplian
ceRegulatoryInformation/PharmacyCompoun
ding/ucm207624.htm

6. American society of plastic surgeons (2008). *ASPS Guiding Principles for Mesotherapy/Injection Lipolysis.* Retrieved from: http://www.plasticsurgery.org/Documents/me dical-professionals/health-policy/guiding-principles/ASPS-Guiding-Principles-for-Mesotherapy-Injection-Lipolysis-7-08.pdf

7. American society for aesthetic plastic surgery (2007). *American Society for Aesthetic Plastic Surgery Warns Patients to Steer Clear of Injection Fat Loss Treatments.* Retrieved from: http://www.surgery.org/media/news-releases/american-society-for-aesthetic-plastic-surgery-warns-patients-to-steer-clear-of-injection-fat-loss-treatment

8. Food and drug administration. *FDA information on lipodissolve* (2010). Retrieved from: http://www.fda.gov/Drugs/GuidanceComplian ceRegulatoryInformation/PharmacyCompoun ding/ucm207624.htm

CHAPTER 9

1. Dr. Robert Kessler, MD. 2121 East Pacific Coast Hwy, Suite 200 Newport Beach, CA 92625 www.drrobkessler.com

CHAPTER 10

1. Baumann, L. (2002). Cosmetic Dermatology: Principals and practice. McGraw-Hill, NY.
2. Thiboutot, D. & Zaenglein, A. (2012) Pathogenesis, clinical manifestations, and diagnosis of acne vulgaris. *Uptodate.com* Retrieved from: http://www.uptodate.com/contents/pathogenes is-clinical-manifestations-and-diagnosis-of-acne-vulgaris?source=see_link
3. Ibid.
4. Baumann, L. (2002). Cosmetic Dermatology: Principals and practice. McGraw-Hill, NY
5. Thiboutot, D. & Zaenglein, A. (2012) Pathogenesis, clinical manifestations, and diagnosis of acne vulgaris. *Uptodate.com* Retrieved from: http://www.uptodate.com/contents/pathogenes is-clinical-manifestations-and-diagnosis-of-acne-vulgaris?source=see_link
6. Baumann, L. (2002). Cosmetic Dermatology: Principals and practice. McGraw-Hill, NY
7. Hatcher, R.A., Trussell, J, Nelson, A. L., Cates, W., Kowal, D. & Policar, M.S. (2011)

Contraceptive technology. (20th ed.): Ardent media

8. Thiboutot, D. & Zaenglein, A. (2012) Pathogenesis, clinical manifestations, and diagnosis of acne vulgaris. *Uptodate.com* Retrieved from: http://www.uptodate.com/contents/pathogenes is-clinical-manifestations-and-diagnosis-of-acne-vulgaris?source=see_link

9. Reszko, A. & Berson, D. (2012) Post-adolescent acne in women. *Uptodate.com* Retrieved from: http://www.uptodate.com/contents/postadolesc ent-acne-in-women?source=search_result&search=acne&s electedTitle=2%7E150#H328490420

10. Baumann, L. (2002). Cosmetic Dermatology: Principals and practice. McGraw-Hill, NY

11. Thiboutot, D. & Zaenglein, A. (2012) Pathogenesis, clinical manifestations, and diagnosis of acne vulgaris. *Uptodate.com* Retrieved from: http://www.uptodate.com/contents/pathogenes is-clinical-manifestations-and-diagnosis-of-acne-vulgaris?source=see_link

12. Ibid.

13. Hatcher, R.A., Trussell, J, Nelson, A. L., Cates, W., Kowal, D. & Policar, M.S. (2011) Contraceptive technology. (20th ed.): Ardent media.

14. Reszko, A. & Berson, D. (2012) Post-adolescent acne in women. *Uptodate.com* Retrieved from: http://www.uptodate.com/contents/postadolesc ent-acne-in-women?source=search_result&search=acne&s electedTitle=2%7E150#H328490420
15. Baumann, L. (2002). Cosmetic Dermatology: Principals and practice. McGraw-Hill, NY
16. Graber, E. (2012). Treatment of Acne Vulgaris *Uptodate.com* Retrieved from: http://www.uptodate.com/contents/treatment-of acnevulgaris?source=search_result&search=ac ne&selectedTitle=1%7E150#H6

CHAPTER 11

1. Taffet, G.E. (2012) Normal aging. Uptodate.com Retrieved from: http://www.uptodate.com/contents/normalagin g?source=preview&anchor=H23810980&sele ctedTitle=36~150#H23810980
2. Ibid.
3. Taffet, G.E. (2012) Normal aging. Uptodate.com Retrieved from: http://www.uptodate.com/contents/normalagin g?source=preview&anchor=H23810980&sele ctedTitle=36~150#H23810980
4. Beckmann, C.R., Ling, F.W., Barzansky, B.M., Herbert, W.N., Laube, D.W., & Smith, R.P. (2010). *Obstetrics and Gynecology: (6ᵗʰ ed.)*. Philadelphia, PA: Lippincott Williams & Wilkins
5. Ibid. 332.

CHAPTER 12

1. Maley, C. (2007). *Your cosmetic practice, a complete guide: What your patients are saying* (pp. 24 & 31). South Carolina: Advantage media group.

About the Author

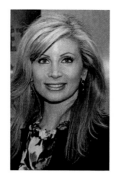

Dr. Beth Haney graduated in 2000 with her Master's degree of Science in Nursing from Loma Linda University and in 2010 earned her Doctorate in Nursing Practice from University of Colorado, Colorado Springs. She has worked in urgent care and family practice as an advanced practice nurse since 2000 and entered the aesthetics industry in 2002. Currently, Dr. Haney holds several positions; Assistant Clinical Professor at University of California, Irvine in the graduate nursing program, clinician at Fullerton College Health Center providing primary care to the student and faculty population, and owner and clinician at Luxe Aesthetic Center in Yorba Linda, CA, specializing in non-surgical cosmetic dermatology.

Dr. Haney also serves on the Board of Directors as President for the California Association for Nurse Practitioners and has held leadership positions in the organization for over 6 years, both at local and state levels. She also sits on a legislative task force for a national association, the American College of Nurse Practitioners, providing legislative information to the leadership and members. She is also an associate of the American Society of Laser Medicine and Surgery, was involved with the Lumenis clinical data collection for a high-speed hair removal laser, and is an international speaker on aesthetics. She lives in Yorba Linda with her husband and two dogs. For more information on Dr. Haney visit her websites at www.luxemedspa.net and www.beyoutfull.net